Wilderness and Rescue Medicine

A Practical Guide

For the Basic and Advanced Practitioner

By Jeffrey E. Isaac, PA-C and David E. Johnson, MD

Erratum: WARM Text

p. 88 Insert at the end of the top paragraph in the right column, "administered as soon as possible after the injury has occurred.

Cleansing the wound usually restarts some bleeding by disturbing the clot. *Do not attempt to clean wounds that are associated with life-threatening bleeding.* Wash the skin around the wound with soap and water and/or a disinfectant like povidone iodine. Clean a wide area of skin, being careful not to allow soap or disinfectant into the wound itself. Irrigate the wound with copious amounts of clean water. Tap water is fine at home. In the field, water filtered or disinfected for drinking is suitable for wound irrigation. When water supplies are limited, using a 1% solution of povidone iodine may reduce the incidence of infection. There is no significant advantage to using sterile saline."

p. 188 Insert after the last sentence on the page, "likely to be on the problem list."

Dedicated to:

John Robert Isaac, MD

Physician, Surgeon, and Father

David would like to thank:
Peter and Jeff
None of this would have been possible without you.

Book design and layout by Dugg Steary

Main mountain photo by Layne Turner
Green tree python photo by Jenny Rollo
Vacuum splint photo by Jeffrey E. Isaac
Sailboat photo by Jean Adam
Helicopter rescue photo by Elvis Santana

Publisher's Note: The information contained in this book is intended to serve as an adjunct to, not a substitute for, professional medical advice and training. The authors disclaim any responsibility for any loss that may occur as a result of information, procedures, or techniques included in this work.

Preface

For nearly 25 years, Wilderness Medical Associates has been teaching practical medicine to people who work in remote and difficult environments. Our core curriculum is designed to provide the skills and insight needed to improvise, adapt, and exercise reasonable judgment at any level of medical training. Although our roots are in the mountains, deserts, and oceans as our name implies, our training philosophy has proven effective in any setting where access to definitive care is delayed or impossible. The term wilderness context applies just as well to a city whose infrastructure has been destroyed as to a fishing boat off the coast of Alaska.

Throughout its history WMA has promoted the idea that pre-hospital practitioners can be trained to make a diagnosis and develop a treatment plan appropriate to whatever challenges they face. The company's founder, Dr. Peter Goth, added spine assessment criteria, the treatment of anaphylaxis, advanced wound care, and other medical protocols to the first aid training of Outward Bound instructors and wilderness guides more than 25 years ago. More importantly, he insisted that his students understand the medical principles behind the procedures. This met with considerable resistance from the mainstream medical community, but was so much more effective than anything previously offered that the program flourished anyway.

Today, wilderness medical training is ubiquitous worldwide, and many of the protocols and training procedures are being adopted by the mainstream emergency medical services. They are learning, as we have, that there is no place in field medicine for unreasonable restrictions on the practical application of medical judgment. This is nowhere more apparent than in a difficult backcountry rescue or the chaos of a mass disaster. We need to give our pre-hospital practitioners the ability to think on their feet and function independently when the medical system is disrupted or unavailable.

Inevitably, we have eliminated some sacred cows and challenged some long-standing assumptions. Double blinded trials, the gold standard for hospital medicine, are few and far between for medicine in the field. Some studies purporting to comprehensively speak for wilderness medicine are too narrowly focused to have much application to the broad range of environments we seek to address. In addition, some of the better-known sources focus on wilderness-related problems but do not pay sufficient attention to the realities of solving them in the field. This is a difficult environment in which to seek scientific validation.

We do not deviate from the mainstream arbitrarily, but are not afraid to do so when necessary. Our opinions and positions are based on careful analysis of the available science and considerable clinical experience, measured against the reality of providing medical care in difficult and dangerous places. We are not trying to change mainstream medicine; we are trying to provide some guidance to those working well outside of it.

We have relied on sources that we believe to be useful enough to at least hint at what may or may not work. This is the interesting and exciting process of extrapolating good science to real field medicine. In doing so, we have applied the collective wisdom of hundreds of instructors, rescue personnel, and medical practitioners. We also owe our grounding in reality, in part, to the contributions and feedback from many of our tens of thousands of graduates.

Nevertheless, Wilderness Medical Associates does not claim to be the final word or the absolute authority on anything. This is a wide-open and rapidly expanding field with a variety of opinions offered by many wise and experienced people. We will continue to offer our own perspective while remaining alert, open, and grateful for the opportunity to learn from others.

David E. Johnson, MD, President
Wilderness Medical Associates

Contents

Section V: Backcountry Medicine

Section VI: Roles and Responsibilities

Section VII: Equipment, Organization, and Materials

Section VIII: Tables and Glossary

Introduction

First and foremost, this book is designed to be a clear, concise, and user-friendly guide to wilderness and rescue medicine. It offers updated material that reflects our knowledge, experience, and the medical literature as of this writing. The content will be appreciated by practitioners at all levels of training but is aimed at the Wilderness First Responder and the Wilderness Emergency Medical Technician. We have also included supplements for advanced practitioners and a bibliography for those seeking more detailed information.

Wilderness and Rescue Medicine is more practical than encyclopedic and is written to be read from front to back. The general principles described in the beginning will enhance your appreciation of the systems and problems discussed later. Your initial understanding of the body systems will guide the process of developing appropriate assessments and treatment plans, and make it easier to gain experience with more complex problems.

Although this text can be understood as a stand-alone resource, it is best accompanied by the WMA Workbook, Lecture Notes, and Field Guide. The case studies that follow some chapters in the text and those in the workbook provide a summary and review of the important principles in a realistic setting, much like the practical sessions during a course. The lecture notes are an expanded version of the same illustrations used in the text, and an abbreviated version of those used in class. Because Wilderness and Rescue Medicine is not designed to be an emergency quick-reference or to be carried in your first aid kit, we offer the Wilderness Medical Associates Field Guide, a smaller, more weather resistant summary of the important information.

Within these publications, you will find certain procedures identified as Wilderness Protocols that define a scope of practice for trained and authorized pre-hospital practitioners. These protocols address specific situations in wilderness and rescue medicine where the procedure clearly exceeds the scope of traditional first aid or emergency medical services practice. Wilderness Medical Associates students are trained and certified in these techniques, but the authorization to use them comes from the practitioner's licensing agency.

The Wilderness Protocols are freely offered for modification and use for the wilderness and rescue setting. Each carries the acknowledgement that the practitioner is appropriately trained and that the protocol is employed only in situations where transport to definitive care would result in unacceptable risk to the patient and/or rescuers. The Wilderness Protocols require a clear diagnosis and a specific action.

Not all situations, however, can be so clearly addressed. As you train for medical care in the unconventional setting, you must be prepared to do some unconventional thinking. Mainstream medical practice may have little relevance to you as the skipper of small boat hundreds of miles from shore or as the leader of rescue team on a high mountain ledge. There are some cases, for example, where applying conventional spine stabilization protocols will substantially increase, rather than decrease, the risk to the patient. For some of you, especially those with years of emergency medical services training, this perspective may be difficult to adopt.

Within the text and presentations, these issues take the form of wilderness context considerations and high-risk problems. You know that the ideal treatment for traumatic brain injury is evacuation to a hospital, but what if the effort will be exceedingly hazardous? How do you balance the risk verses the potential benefit? These types of decisions are not easy, but they are necessary.

This text and the courses it serves are designed to provide you with some background with which to make tough choices and to provide the most effective medical care possible in unique and challenging circumstances. In addition to understanding principles and learning procedures, you will need to keep an open mind. The ability to innovate and adapt will serve you far better than trying to memorize a protocol for every circumstance.

Finally, if you are new to the study of medicine, you may feel overwhelmed by abbreviations, mnemonics and acronyms. Even experienced practitioners are occasionally baffled by their colleague's documentation shortcuts. To help with some of this, we have included a glossary and list of abbreviations in the back of the text. No doubt, we have missed many of them and will continue to add new ones to future editions of this book. Detailed information about drugs mentioned within the text can also be found here.

All of us at Wilderness Medical Associates hope that you find Wilderness and Rescue Medicine interesting, relevant, and useful. We plan to update and revise this text and our curriculum frequently, and we welcome and encourage your comments and critique. The authors can be reached through Wilderness Medical Associates, 400 Riverside Street, Suite A6, Portland, ME USA 04103. E-mail: office@wildmed.com. Web: www.wildmed.com.

Section I

General Principles and Patient Assessment

General Principles of Physiology and Pathology

Most emergency medical diagnoses and treatments, however sophisticated, are based on a few general principles of pathology and physiology. By understanding these basic features of human response to injury and illness, you will be in a much better position to adapt medical treatment to the remote or extreme environment. Training in specific skills is certainly important, but if you can truly understand the principles behind the procedures, you will never forget what to do. You will understand what needs to be done. These principles are fundamental, easily understood, and will surface frequently in your study and practice of wilderness and rescue medicine.

OXYGENATION AND PERFUSION

All living tissue must be continuously perfused with oxygenated blood to function and survive. For each cell in the body to be adequately oxygenated requires a continuous flow of fresh air to the lungs and a continuous flow of blood to the body tissues. Anything that interferes with this is a serious problem. The preservation of oxygenation and perfusion is the primary purpose of emergency medical care.

The primary function of the respiratory system is to bring outside air into the alveoli of the lungs where

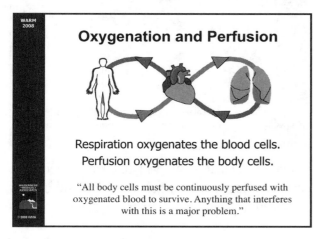

Oxygenation and Perfusion

Respiration oxygenates the blood cells.
Perfusion oxygenates the body cells.

"All body cells must be continuously perfused with oxygenated blood to survive. Anything that interferes with this is a major problem."

only a thin membrane separates air from blood. This allows oxygen from the air to enter the blood and combine with hemoglobin in red blood cells and for excess carbon dioxide to diffuse from the blood into the air. Adequate oxygenation of the blood requires adequate respiration.

The function of the circulatory system is to perfuse body tissues with oxygenated blood. Adequate perfusion requires that the circulatory system generates enough pressure to force the blood through the miles of tiny capillaries where oxygenation of the cells and removal of metabolic waste occurs.

THREE CRITICAL BODY SYSTEMS, THREE MAJOR PROBLEMS

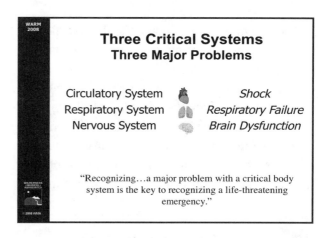

Three Critical Systems
Three Major Problems

Circulatory System — Shock
Respiratory System — Respiratory Failure
Nervous System — Brain Dysfunction

"Recognizing…a major problem with a critical body system is the key to recognizing a life-threatening emergency."

The organs of the circulatory, respiratory, and nervous systems perform the functions most essential to life. A major problem with any one of these three systems represents an immediate threat to life. Your initial patient assessment is designed to quickly evaluate the essential functions of these three systems.

The term shock indicates inadequate perfusion pressure in the circulatory system resulting in inadequate tissue oxygenation. Inadequate oxygenation of the blood by the respiratory system is termed respiratory failure. Anything that impairs brain function can inhibit control and function of the other two critical systems.

These three critical systems are interdependent. A problem with one will quickly affect the functions of the other two. For example: shock from blood loss will stimulate an increase in the respiratory rate and cause changes in mental status. Because the critical systems affect each other in a variety of ways, it can be a challenge to determine in which critical system the original problem lies.

Coordinated function of the circulatory, respiratory, and nervous systems is required to maintain adequate oxygenation and perfusion. Recognizing or anticipating the development of a major problem with a critical body system is the key to recognizing a life-threatening emergency. This skill is equally helpful in recognizing when you don't have an emergency, which is most of the time.

COMPENSATION

The nervous system regulates the function of the circulatory and respiratory systems to maintain adequate oxygenation and perfusion under a variety of conditions. The brain compensates for the effects of an injury or illness by adjusting cardiac output, respiratory rate and effort, and tissue perfusion.

We measure compensation mechanisms and their effects by checking vital signs: pulse rate, respiratory rate and effort, level of consciousness and mental status, blood pressure, skin perfusion, and body core temperature. Minor changes will occur as the healthy body adapts to the various stresses of normal life. A pattern of substantial, progressive, or persistent changes in vital signs indicates an evolving problem. Observing the pattern and progression of vital sign changes is the best way to detect the development of a critical system problem in its early stages. The volume shock pattern shown is a good example.

THE EVOLUTIONARY ONION

Nervous system tissue, including the brain, is exquisitely sensitive to oxygen deprivation and will often exhibit the earliest signs and symptoms of a problem with oxygenation and perfusion. The severity of these symptoms correlates well to the severity of the problem. We measure these effects in our assessment of mental status and level of consciousness.

Picture the brain as a sort of onion with increasingly complex layers of function from the inside out. The basic physiologic functions such as vasoconstriction, heart rate, and respiratory rate extend from the innermost and more primitive layers in the brain stem. Higher brain function, such as personality, judgment, and problem solving are controlled by the outer layers of the brain. These outer layers are also the first to be affected when problems develop.

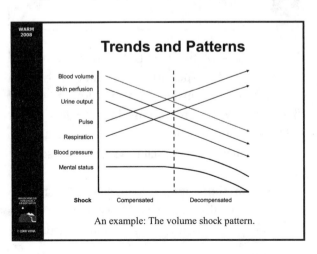

An example: The volume shock pattern.

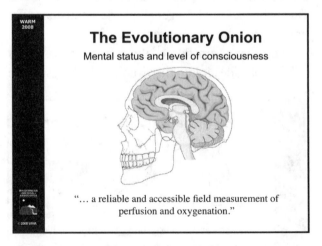

Altered mental status will often be the earliest vital sign change seen when perfusion and cellular oxygenation is impaired. Patients remain conscious and alert, but may become anxious, uncooperative, or respond in ways that do not fit the situation. They may act belligerent or confused. WMA students often use the phrase "peeling the onion" to describe this condition.

More extreme problems affect the deeper layers of the brain and cause a decrease in level of consciousness. When the onion has peeled this far, the situation has become much more serious. The progression can also be reversed if the underlying problems are corrected. Monitoring consciousness and mental status offers a reliable and accessible field measurement of the quality of oxygenation and perfusion.

SWELLING AND PRESSURE

Swelling is caused by the accumulation of excess fluid in body tissues. It can develop quickly as blood escapes from ruptured arteries, or slowly as serum oozes from damaged or inflamed capillaries, causing the condition known as edema. It may be localized, like the swelling of a sprained ankle, or systemic, like the swelling of the whole body that occurs in allergic reactions.

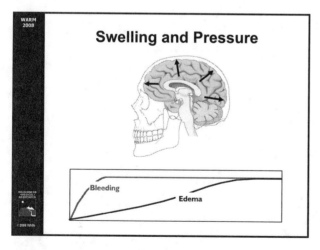

Swelling is annoying when it causes pain and dangerous when it causes problems with perfusion and oxygenation. Swelling that develops inside a restricted space such as the skull or a muscle compartment can result in enough pressure to restrict perfusion, causing the condition known as ischemia.

This is exactly what happens to the brain with the development of increased intracranial pressure due to head injury. It is also responsible for the damage caused by a compartment syndrome that develops in the lower leg or forearm. Swelling in the confined space of the upper airway can cause obstruction, while swelling lower in the respiratory system can cause lower airway constriction or pulmonary edema.

Most of the swelling that occurs following injury develops during the first 24 hours. Swelling will increase very little thereafter unless there is repeat injury or persistent inflammation. Anticipating and controlling the development of swelling is essential to the preservation of oxygenation and perfusion, and the prevention of ischemia and necrosis. If significant swelling does not develop within 24 hours, it is unlikely that it will.

ISCHEMIA TO INFARCTION

Inadequate local tissue perfusion is called ischemia. This is distinguished from the term shock, which is used to describe inadequate systemic perfusion. Symptoms of ischemia include pain and impaired function. The chest pain of a heart attack, for example, is caused by ischemia of heart muscle.

Prolonged ischemia will inevitably lead to infarction, which is the term for tissue death (also called necrosis). Some tissue, like the brain, will die within a few minutes. The skin, however, can live for hours without adequate perfusion. It seems that the more important an organ is to immediate survival the more sensitive it is to the loss of perfusion.

Ischemia can be complete or partial. It can develop from an internal problem such as a blood clot or compartment syndrome, or from external pressure such as a tight splint or laying on an unpadded backboard. The symptoms of ischemia are an early warning of the serious and permanent problems caused by infarction.

OBSTRUCTION TO INFECTION

The human body is full of hollow organs that store, transport, or excrete liquids of all types. These include sweat glands, intestines, bladder, and all of the associated ducts. If the drainage from these organs is obstructed by swelling, deformity, or a foreign body, the accumulation and pressure will cause inflammation and pain. If the obstruction lasts long enough, any bacteria present will begin to grow out of control in whatever substance is trapped and infection will develop. The most common example is the average pimple. This is an infection in an obstructed sweat gland. Appendicitis is another example of the same principle, just a bit more serious. Many illnesses have their origins in obstruction.

NOTES:

General Principles of Wilderness Rescue

2

An experienced rescuer will have learned not to expect a predictable and comfortable work environment. Flexibility, innovation, and a certain amount of courage are required to cope with the varied and constantly evolving nature of medical care in the wild or remote setting. There are, however, a few guiding principles and practices that can help to impose some degree of order on chaos. These are the general principles of wilderness rescue.

THE RISK/BENEFIT RATIO

There are countless examples of high-risk solutions to low-risk medical problems. This is nowhere more apparent than in backcountry and marine rescue. The reasons are not difficult to understand: incomplete medical information, emotional involvement in the patient's plight, and the excitement and allure of the rescue operation itself.

Every treatment (or decision not to treat) and every emergency evacuation (or decision to stay in the field) involves the risk that the medical problems will become worse because of what we've done. We also run the risk of causing injury to the rescuers themselves or to other people that may be involved. Against this risk, we balance the potential benefits

The Risk/Benefit Ratio

Avoid high-risk solutions to low-risk problems!

"Good decisions reflect the clear assessment that the benefit outweighs the risk."

of our actions. Good decisions reflect the clear assessment that the benefit outweighs the risk.

Risk/benefit decisions can be considered a form of medical judgment usually reserved for licensed practitioners. In the wilderness setting, judgment becomes a required skill at any level of medical training. It is often up to the person in charge of medical care on scene to convey the appropriate sense of urgency, determine the type of care needed next, and figure out how to access it safely and efficiently.

THE BIG MAGNIFIER

Risk is a function of both probability and consequence. While the probability of becoming injured or ill in remote settings may be no greater than on the street, the consequences can be far worse. The blister that goes unmentioned on the hike into camp can become a debilitating infection that prevents escape from an approaching storm.

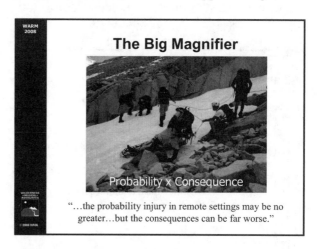

The Big Magnifier

Probability x Consequence

"…the probability injury in remote settings may be no greater…but the consequences can be far worse."

Frostbitten fingers become useless when rewarmed, keeping the patient from handling skis or ice tools. You might have no higher a probability of a slip and fall on the top of a snowfield in the mountains than while walking to the post office in town, but it is the consequence that makes the difference. This important principle reminds us that prevention and early intervention is the prime duty for the wilderness medical practitioner. Whenever possible, avoid the combination of high probability and high consequence.

THE PROBLEM LIST

Practitioners familiar with the SOAP format for medical documentation will recognize the problem list as the A, or assessment. This is how you render order from chaos. Constructing a succinct list of problems identified by the scene survey and examination of the patient begins a well-ordered process of treatment and evacuation. For each problem identified, a priority is established and a treatment is planned. The problem list is also your primary tool for communicating the patient's condition and treatment to other people.

In the wilderness or disaster setting, the patient's medical condition may be just a small part of a much larger problem list that includes adverse weather, difficult terrain, and hazardous working conditions. These factors can create new medical problems as well as determine the plan for dealing with the existing ones. For the wilderness medical practitioner, the problem list includes the environmental issues along with the medical.

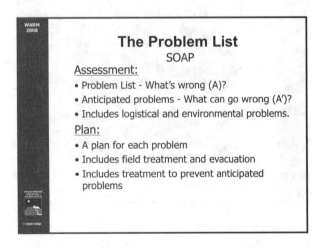

GENERIC TO SPECIFIC

In medical practice, the process of diagnosis moves from generic to specific, with the treatment and referral following suit. But, if your examining room is the salon of a small boat 200 miles offshore, getting more than a general idea of the patient's problem may not be possible. The practitioner is often left working with a generic diagnosis for the duration of field treatment and evacuation.

The differential diagnosis of abdominal pain, for example, is a long and complicated list. Without x-ray, ultrasound, and laboratory, it is nearly impossible for the examiner to distinguish an ectopic pregnancy from appendicitis or any one of a dozen other surgical emergencies. Fortunately, the generic diagnosis of serious abdominal pain is all that is necessary to make an appropriate field treatment decision. This patient needs a hospital, and your job is supportive care and

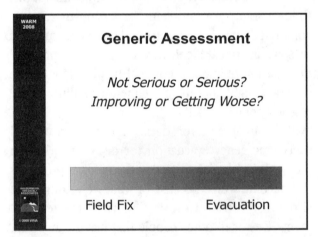

urgent evacuation. You don't want to waste a lot of time trying to put a specific name on something you can't treat in the field, anyway.

THE BIG NET

A corollary to the generic-to-specific principle is the need to consider and treat all likely and possible causes of a problem until a specific diagnosis and treatment can be rendered, especially when a critical body system is involved. Altered mental status in a high-altitude climber could be caused by HAPE, hypothermia, hypoxia, intoxication, brain injury, or low blood sugar.

The practitioner considers all of these potential causes initially, including them on the working problem list and treating them accordingly. As further investigation is done and the results of treatment are observed, some of the possible causes can be ruled out and the treatment directed at those that are left.

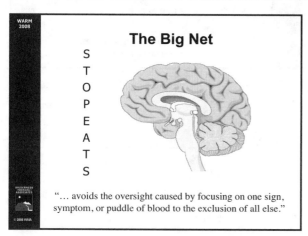

Casting the Big Net avoids the oversight caused by puddle vision, that is, inappropriately focusing on one sign, symptom, or puddle of blood to the exclusion of all else.

IDEAL TO REAL

Medical practitioners are fond of the excuse "if I just had my jump kit, or nurse, or defibrillator. . ." In a wilderness rescue situation, you are not being quizzed on the ideal hospital or clinic treatment for the condition you've identified. You are being challenged to come up with a plan that makes sense for the environment in which you are operating.

It is certainly helpful to have the ideal treatment in mind, but you must be able to forgive yourself for not being able to provide it. In some cases, you may be able to come close. In most cases, you will have to accept compromise and be willing to execute a plan that is "real" for the situation the patient is in.

For example, the ideal treatment for a trauma patient with neck pain might involve spine stabilization with a cervical collar and vacuum mattress. But if your problem list includes being 20 meters down a crevasse in an Antarctic glacier, your patient may freeze to death before this can be accomplished. Helping the patient climb out may be the only real treatment for a situation like this.

"THE PATIENT IS THE ONE WITH THE DISEASE"

This time-honored medical school quip is another way of saying, "Don't panic." The acute stress reaction caused by a crisis is perfectly normal but rarely helpful. To settle your own emotions, remember that you are not the one injured and in need of help. You are help.

You will function more efficiently and safely by remaining objective and task-oriented. The more confusing and complicated the problem, the more important this behavior is. This can take considerable self-discipline.

Rescue scenes are full of distractions courtesy of radio traffic, bystanders, fellow rescuers, and anyone suffering pain and acute stress reaction. Your attention will be drawn in a dozen different directions. Learn to focus your attention on the problems that are truly urgent and important, and those that are going to be urgent and important if you don't do something about them. Avoid addressing anything that is not important to the care and safety of your patient and crew. To an untrained or uninformed observer, you may appear detached or overly concerned with your own safety. Their perceptions are not your problem; the conduct of a safe and competent rescue is.

MEDICINE IS DYNAMIC

Everything in medicine, from general principles of care to specific treatment, carries some degree of uncertainty. Fortunately, some of what we do is validated by extensive experience and good science. But, we must remember that our practice setting bears little resemblance to the conditions under which most medical studies are performed.

Although laboratory science and medical center

practice has plenty to teach us, it must be measured against the irreducible reality of providing care in a remote and dangerous place. Some of our practices and protocols are still based on anecdotal experience and incomplete scientific evidence. Where even less experience is available, we still rely on educated speculation supported only by what seems to make sense. As more data becomes available, some widely accepted medical practices will be debunked and others validated. Medical practitioners at every level of training must be willing to reevaluate the standard of care whenever new information and field experience suggests a better way. We should be prepared to improvise, adapt, and keep an open mind.

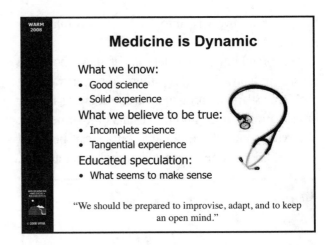

NOTES:

The Patient Assessment System

The Patient Assessment System (PAS) is a tool for organized response to any situation. Properly applied, it will lead you to a concise description of the problems with which you are dealing and what you're going to do about them. The ultimate desired result is called the problem list and plan. The more confused and difficult the situation is, the more valuable a well-rehearsed PAS will be. This is the way to impose order on chaos.

The PAS consists of three important steps: gathering information, creating a problem list, and planning treatment and evacuation. Information is collected in a series of surveys, which is summarized as three triangles. This information can then organized in a format abbreviated as SOAP—Subjective, Objective, Assessment, and Plan. Most medical professionals use this system in one form or another.

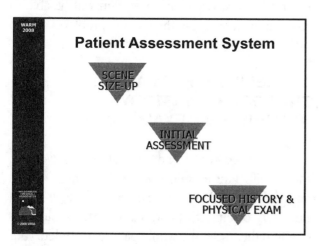

GATHERING INFORMATION: THE SCENE SIZE-UP

The scene size-up will keep you alive and functioning. It also serves to protect other rescuers, bystanders, and the patient from further harm. If you are among the first on scene, a complete scene size-up is your first responsibility.

It can take tremendous discipline to overcome the urge to rush to the aid of a person in trouble, but this is exactly what you must do. Stop, look around, and identify hazards to yourself and your team. The threats may be environmental like frigid water or a hang-fire avalanche, or generated by the activities of other people. Whatever it is, if it can harm you or your fellow rescuers, it must be stabilized before you can do anything else.

Included in this survey of dangers is the potential for exposure to body fluids. A number of diseases can be transmitted via body fluids, including HIV and Hepatitis. The use of universal precautions is now standard in all areas of medicine where body fluid contact is possible. This includes using gloves, eye protection, face masks, hand washing, antiseptics and proper disposal techniques.

Once you are safe, or relatively so, look for any further threat to bystanders and the injured person. Stabilize the scene by moving danger from the patient

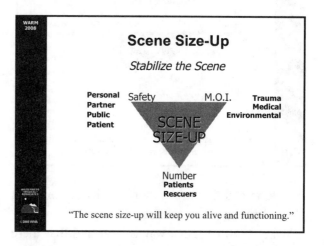

or the patient from the danger. This has priority over everything else that follows. So, get him out of the water or out from under the cornice and clear the area of well-meaning but unsafe people.

As you do this, try to evaluate the mechanism of injury. How the problem developed is usually obvious, but occasionally more investigation will be necessary. For example, how far did he fall? Was it enough of a tumble to cause significant injury? Are there other factors such as exposure to weather that might contribute to the patient's condition?

Your scene survey also determines how many people are injured or at risk. This is especially important in harsh environments where all field personnel may be at risk for hypothermia or dehydration. In mass casualty situations, more seriously injured people are often overlooked in the rush to treat the most noisy and uncomfortable patients.

GATHERING INFORMATION: THE INITIAL ASSESSMENT

The initial assessment is your quick-check on the status of the patient's three critical body systems. The circulatory, respiratory, and nervous systems are equally important to survival, and their associated major problems are equally life threatening. The order in which you check and stabilize them should

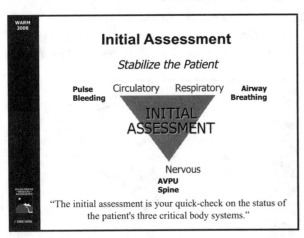

be determined by the situation, not by the order in which they appear on any list.

Make sure that the airway is clear and that there is sufficient respiratory effort to oxygenate the lungs. Check for the presence of a pulse, and determine if it seems fast, slow, or normal. Perform a quick exam for severe bleeding. While you are doing this, try to

ensure that the patient's spine is stable, and assess the level of consciousness.

Your initial assessment might be as simple as asking, "How do you do?" and getting a "fine" and a smile. Or, you might be on belay in a crevasse listening for breath sounds and looking inside bulky clothing for blood. Whatever form it takes, it is a critical step in your organized approach to the situation. Any problems encountered in the initial assessment must be immediately stabilized before worrying about anything else. Do not become distracted by messy or painful injuries like deformed fractures and bloody abrasions. Distraction can keep you from finding the urgent and important problems like airway obstruction or severe bleeding.

The immediate hands-on management of life-threatening problems found in the initial assessment is referred to as basic life support (BLS), and includes cardiopulmonary resuscitation (CPR). Advanced Life Support (ALS) adds medications and specialized tools to manage these same critical system problems. You may not get any further than BLS or ALS with your assessment and treatment if the injury or illness is severe. In most cases, however, you will be able to rule out or stabilize life-threatening problems and go on to the focused history and physical exam.

GATHERING INFORMATION: THE FOCUSED HISTORY AND PHYSICAL EXAM

The focused history and physical exam is a slower, more deliberate examination of the patient. Speed and detail will change with circumstance. It is not necessary or efficient to stop and treat problems as you find them. Get the whole picture, complete your list, and then return to treat each problem in order of priority.

Most practitioners are accustomed to patients sitting quietly on an exam table and like to start with the head and neck and then move to the chest, abdomen, pelvis, legs, arms, and back. It's comforting to have a routine. It can keep the examiner on task even when he's distracted by thoughts of sailing or hiking or being anywhere but the office.

A well-rehearsed routine will be even more valuable in the backcountry situation while you're distracted by wind, cold, radio traffic, and thoughts of being anywhere but this mountainside. You may not yet know what the problem is, but you know what to do: examine the patient. The PAS will focus your attention and lead to a plan.

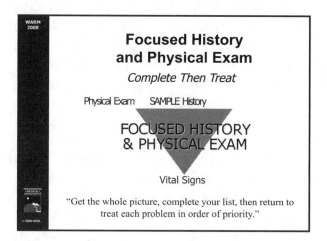

**Focused History
and Physical Exam**

Complete Then Treat

Physical Exam   SAMPLE History

FOCUSED HISTORY
& PHYSICAL EXAM

Vital Signs

"Get the whole picture, complete your list, then return to treat each problem in order of priority."

Your exam should be as comprehensive as the situation requires and allows. Realistically, the order in which you perform your exam makes no difference. Start where it makes sense to start. If the patient is lying face down, examine the back first. It is not necessary to see or feel every body part in every patient. If no symptom or mechanism of injury suggests involvement, exposure and examination is not important in the field. It is important that the rescuer go through a complete head to toe checklist, mentally if not physically.

The complaint of a sprained thumb by an otherwise healthy person does not warrant a complete survey with vital signs and a detailed physical exam. But, a person with altered mental status and a mechanism for significant injury certainly does. The less information the patient is able to give you, the more information you will need from your exam.

Your detailed exam catalogs anything abnormal such as tenderness, discoloration, swelling, and deformity. You don't have to be an experienced anatomist to recognize a deformed long bone or the

fact that the abdomen is rigid when it is supposed to be soft. If your patient is at all responsive, you will be able to find out what hurts.

Advanced practitioners will listen for breath sounds with a stethoscope, look in ears, and peer down throats. The abdominal exam might also include listening to bowel sounds and palpating for organ enlargement. The neurological exam may be as simple as talking to the patient to determine mental status, or as complete as testing all twelve cranial nerves and deep tendon reflexes. The complexity of your exam will depend on your level of comfort and training. In all but the simplest case, any exam is better than no exam.

In an unresponsive or unreliable patient, your exam might also include the patient's pockets or pack. A medication bottle, insulin syringe, or medic alert bracelet can provide valuable information in a confusing case. Respect privacy, but get the data that you need.

VITAL SIGNS

While the initial assessment looks quickly for urgent problems, the measurement of vital signs provides a more complete view of critical system function and compensation. Decay or improvement will be revealed by changes in the vital sign pattern over time. This can serve to reassure you that the patient is okay or provide an early warning of developing trouble. The detail with which you measure vital signs will depend on the equipment available and your level of training. How often you measure vital signs will depend on the logistical situation and your level of comfort with the patient's condition.

Pulse (P) is easy to measure accurately and reflects almost any change in the circulatory system. Pulse rate is expressed in beats per minute, and can be quickly obtained by counting the pulse for 15 seconds and multiplying by four. Noting the rhythm (irregular or regular) can be helpful in some cases, but subjective assessments like weak, thready, or bounding are rarely useful. You can find the pulse in any artery, but the radial (wrist), carotid (neck), and temporal (temple) are the most accessible.

Respiratory rate (R), expressed in breaths per minute, is a direct measurement of respiratory system function but can be difficult to measure accurately. It is more valuable to note the effort involved in respiration. An increased respiratory rate may actually be a compensatory response to shock, which is a circulatory system problem. But, labored and noisy respiration would confirm a respiratory system

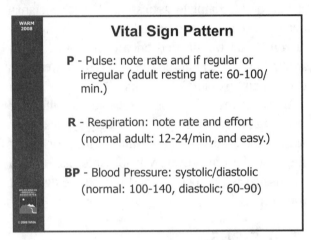

Vital Sign Pattern

P - Pulse: note rate and if regular or irregular (adult resting rate: 60-100/min.)

R - Respiration: note rate and effort (normal adult: 12-24/min, and easy.)

BP - Blood Pressure: systolic/diastolic (normal: 100-140, diastolic; 60-90)

problem and true respiratory distress.

Blood Pressure (BP), like pulse, is a measurement of circulatory system function. A reading of 120/80 would be typical for an adult. The systolic reading indicates the pressure produced by the force of each heart contraction. The diastolic reading reflects the resting pressure of the system maintained by arterial muscle tone. The systolic pressure is the most useful and the easiest to measure in the emergency setting.

Systolic BP is usually measured by inflating a blood pressure cuff around the arm and applying enough pressure to completely stop arterial blood flow. The cuff is then slowly deflated while the examiner watches the gauge and feels for the return of a pulse in the wrist. The reading on the gauge when the first beat is felt is the systolic BP. Diastolic BP is obtained by listening to arterial flow with a stethoscope or Doppler device. Automated BP cuffs capable of measuring systolic and diastolic are often used in ambulances and emergency departments. As these devices become smaller and more reliable, they are appearing in the jumps kits used by ski patrols and backcountry rescue teams.

Temperature (T) refers to the temperature of the body core. This can be quite different from skin temperature, even in the normal patient. The rectum is the most accurate place to easily measure core temperature in the field. Oral temperatures are certainly more convenient, but affected by eating, breathing, and talking. Readings will usually be about a degree lower than core temperature. The more accurate esophageal and tympanic probes are generally not available or practical for field use.

Skin (S) color and temperature reflects the perfusion of the body shell. Reduced skin perfusion may indicate compensation for loss of blood volume in illness and injury. Or, cool and pale skin might just be part of the normal response to cold weather. Warm, dry, and pink is normal. The perfusion status of dark skinned patients can be assessed by observing the palms and soles, and mucosa of the lips.

Consciousness and Mental Status (C/MS) is a measure of brain function. No special instruments

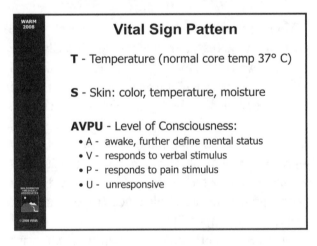

Vital Sign Pattern

T - Temperature (normal core temp 37° C)

S - Skin: color, temperature, moisture

AVPU - Level of Consciousness:
• A - awake, further define mental status
• V - responds to verbal stimulus
• P - responds to pain stimulus
• U - unresponsive

are required. Consciousness is described as relating to one of four letters on the AVPU scale. A is used to describe the condition of being awake or alert. The patient who is awake is further described in terms of mental status using terms like oriented, disoriented, confused, combative, and so on. A patient who is V on AVPU appears unaware but responds to verbal stimulus. The response may range from actually answering a question to just a grunt or turn of the head. P indicates a response only to pain. The patient may localize to pain by pushing your hand away from an injury or respond with just a groan or non-specific movement. A patient who is U does not respond to anything.

When measuring vital signs, it is most useful to take all six together at regular intervals allowing you to observe change over time. Even without blood pressure cuffs, clinical thermometers, or a watch, a valuable assessment of vital signs can still be made. Measurements become relative: Pulse is "fast" or "slow;" temperature is "cool" or "warm." Blood pressure can be assessed as "normal" or "low" based on signs like mental status and skin color.

SAMPLE HISTORY

History can be gathered before or after the physical exam. Beware of the common mistake of taking a history while performing the exam. "Does this hurt?" and "Have you ever had abdominal surgery?" asked at the same time may produce a useless answer to both questions. In the ideal situation, your history will be gathered separately.

The history should be focused like the exam. Details about your patient's abdominal surgery in 1983 are not relevant to the assessment of his sprained knee. But, the history of surgery would certainly be relevant in evaluating a complaint of abdominal pain because surgical scars can increase the risk of bowel obstruction.

A history of allergy is especially important if you are thinking of giving medication. Questions about last

food and fluids are important where extreme weather is an issue or if you suspect volume shock from dehydration. The events question pertains specifically to what happened that directly led to the problem with which you are dealing. This could be a description of a fall, a long hike leading to heat exhaustion, or being stung by a wasp. Careful attention here can reveal undiscovered problems or help make the difference between diagnosing a critical system problem like a traumatic brain injury, and reassuring yourself that you're looking at a simple scalp contusion. A good history is often the most useful part of the whole assessment process.

CREATING A PROBLEM LIST—SOAP

The information you've gathered in your surveys is organized in a format abbreviated SOAP: Subjective, Objective, Assessment, and Plan. It provides the answer to the all-important question: What are you going to do with this patient? It is the way medical records are written and the way medical information is communicated. The general meaning of each heading is:

S - Subjective: Description of the scene, the mechanism of injury, symptoms that the patient is complaining about, and relevant history (SAMPLE).

O - Objective: What you see, hear, feel, and smell during your

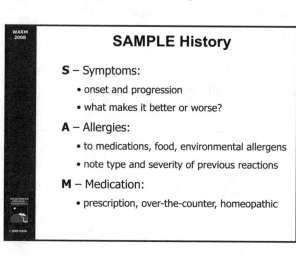

SAMPLE History

S – Symptoms:
  • onset and progression
  • what makes it better or worse?
A – Allergies:
  • to medications, food, environmental allergens
  • note type and severity of previous reactions
M – Medication:
  • prescription, over-the-counter, homeopathic

SAMPLE History

P – Pertinent History:
  • Previous similar symptoms or problems
  • Contributing factors
L – Last Ins and Outs:
  • Food, fluids: time and quantity
  • Urine and bowel, normal or abnormal
E – Events:
  • Leading up to the accident or illness
  • Consider mixed mechanisms

examination of the patient, including vital signs.

A - Assessment: The concise problem list based on the subjective and objective findings. It also includes anticipated problems (A') that may develop as a result of existing problems or environmental conditions.

P - Plan: What you are going to do about each problem, including medical treatments, plans for monitoring the patient's condition, and plans for evacuation.

EXAMPLE:

Using this system, a typical brief SOAP for an emergency room case might look like this:

S: A 19-year-old man fell off his bicycle when he rode over a curb at slow speed. He complains of pain in his right wrist and tingling of his fingers. He has no complaints of pain anywhere else. He was not wearing a helmet, but did not hit his head and has full memory for the event. No allergies, no medications, no past history of wrist injury, last meal 12:00.

O: An alert, oriented, but uncomfortable man. The right wrist is swollen and tender to touch. There is no other obvious injury. The patient refuses to move the wrist voluntarily. The fingers are warm and pink and can be wiggled with slight pain felt at the wrist. The patient can feel the light touch of a cotton swab on the end of each finger. X-Ray shows a buckle fracture of the distal radius.
VS: P: 80. R: 18, easy. BP: 122/72. S: w/d/p. T: 37.1° centigrade. C: Awake, alert, and oriented.

A: Fracture right wrist.

P: Wrist splint. Rest, ice, and elevation. Ibuprofen 800 mg every 8 hours for pain. Follow up with an orthopedic surgeon in 3 days. Return to the hospital if fingers become blue or cold, or the tingling becomes at all worse.

This format paints a nice picture of the situation. In just a few words, you get a sense for who the patient is and what happened, and what the practitioner is going to do about it. There is also a brief description of problems that might develop and what the patient's response should be.

The SOAP format is perfectly adaptable to the backcountry setting. It performs the same vital function that it does in the emergency department. SOAP organizes your thoughts and allows you to communicate your ideas and plans.

EXAMPLE:

Now, let's take this same case into the backcountry:

S: A 19-year-old man fell over the handlebars on a mountain bike ride near Horse Thief Canyon about one hour ago. He complains of pain in his right wrist and tingling of his fingers. He has no complaints of pain anywhere else. He did not hit his head and has full memory for the event. No allergies, no medications, no past history of wrist injury, last meal 12:00. He feels cold and hungry.

It is now 18:30 and getting dark. The air temperature is 48°. It is raining lightly. The scene is a three-hour bike ride from the trailhead.

O: At 18:30: An alert, responsive but uncomfortable man is found sitting on a rock holding his right arm. He is cool, wet, and inadequately dressed. His right wrist is slightly swollen and tender to touch, and he is unable to move it. He can wiggle his fingers and feel the light touch of the examiner's hand. His skin color is pale. There is no other obvious injury.

VS: P: 80. R: 18, easy. BP 122 systolic. S: cool and pale. T: 37.1° centigrade. C: Awake and oriented.

A: 1. Unstable injury right wrist.
　　　　　A': swelling and ischemia
　　　　　A': pain
　　　　2. Cold response.
　　　　　A': hypothermia
　　　　3. Dark, wet, unsafe riding or hiking conditions.

P: 1. Wrist splint. Elevation and rest. Ibuprofen. Monitor distal CSM.
　　　　2. Dry clothes, food, and shelter from the rain and wind.
　　　　3. Stay on-scene tonight, walk out tomorrow.

You can see that we need to expand SOAP to include environmental and logistical factors. We must consider problems created by weather, terrain, distance, and time. Sometimes these are more of a threat than the original injury or illness. In long-term care, we also add a list of "anticipated problems" (A') which could be complications of the injury itself or the result of exposure to environmental conditions.

In this example, the anticipated problem of hypothermia is included because it often occurs in wet and cool weather, especially in a person who is not exercising and eating well. By listing it as a potential problem, we are reminded to take measures to prevent it. This is a perfect use for the anticipated problem list.

In more complicated cases where a patient may

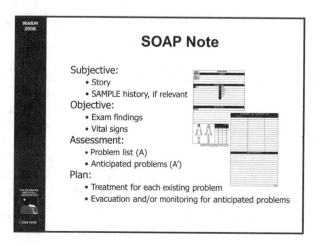

have more than one problem, the format remains the same. Under A (Assessment), we would list the problems in order of priority, and be sure that we have a plan for each one. By checking each problem for a plan and each plan for a problem, we can avoid missing anything. We can also avoid making plans for problems that don't exist.

As our patient's condition and evacuation logistics change, our problem list and plans will need to be revised. Backcountry rescue is rarely straightforward and predictable. Monitoring the condition of the

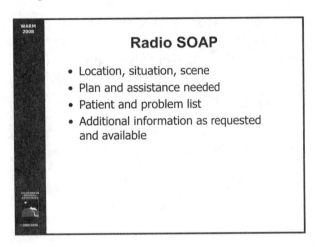

Radio SOAP

- Location, situation, scene
- Plan and assistance needed
- Patient and problem list
- Additional information as requested and available

patient and crew is essential. SOAP is a dynamic process.

Patients with anticipated critical body system problems should be reassessed most often, at least every 15 minutes, if possible. The status of injured extremities in a reliable patient can be checked less frequently at one to two hour intervals. Conditions which develop slowly, such as wound infection, might be adequately monitored every six hours.

Our problems list also becomes a useful communication tool when we're trying to conserve radio batteries or quickly update other rescuers arriving on-scene. "Unstable right wrist, cold response" gives the relevant information in just a few words. You can imagine how useful this might be in a mass casualty incident or other high-stress operation.

When time and batteries allow, more complete information can be relayed. Still, the practitioner will want to keep the message concise. The essential points can be lost in too much information.

Try to paint a picture of your situation, including your problem list and plan. "This is Search and Rescue on the scene of a mountain bike accident mile 42, White Rim Trail. One male patient; problems are unstable right wrist and cold response. Weather is cold rain and wind. We will stay here tonight and evacuate in the morning." In this case, relaying vital signs and negative findings is unnecessary. The receiving station knows your situation, problem list, and plan.

NOTES:

Section II

Critical Body Systems and Life Support

The Circulatory System

4

STRUCTURE AND FUNCTION

For field purposes, we can consider the structure of the circulatory system to consist of three basic components: the blood, the blood vessels, and the heart. They work together to distribute oxygen and nutrients and to remove waste.

The blood serves as the primary transport medium and is composed of fluid, cells, and dissolved gasses. The fluid component of the blood consists of water, proteins, electrolytes, and the various chemical mediators of body function called hormones. The cellular component includes red blood cells to carry oxygen, white blood cells to fight infection, and platelets to effect blood clotting.

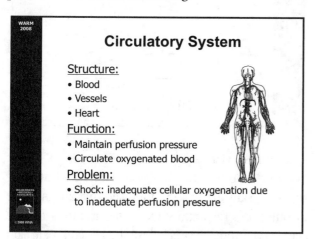

The average human body contains about five liters of blood; however, this volume is not contained in a closed system. The fluid component can migrate between the interior of body cells, the space between the cells, and the blood itself. These three fluid spaces are called the intracellular space, the extracellular space, and the vascular space. This ability to shift fluid explains how a patient can lose blood volume by losing water and electrolytes from sweat glands. It also explains how blood volume can be restored by drinking water and electrolytes.

The blood serves all living cells in the body (with the exception of the cornea of the eye) by traveling within a system of arteries, veins, and capillaries. There are two zones in the system, one circulating through the lungs and the other through the rest of the body. The former allows for oxygenation of the blood, the latter for oxygenation of the body cells.

As the blood is pumped from the right ventricle of the heart it flows into the pulmonary circulation in the lungs, where oxygenation of the blood occurs and carbon dioxide is released to be exhaled. Oxygenated blood returning from the lungs enters the left side of the heart where the left ventricle pumps it to the rest of the body. From the thoracic aorta, which is about the diameter of a garden hose, the blood flows through progressively smaller vessels into the capillary beds. These consist of a dense matrix of vessels about the diameter of a red blood cell. This is how blood is brought into very close proximity to individual body cells, allowing for cellular oxygenation and the removal of carbon dioxide. Exiting the capillaries, the blood enters the veins to be returned to the right side of the heart.

To keep you alive, your five liters of blood is pumped through approximately fourteen kilometers of blood vessels about a thousand times per day. Considerable pressure is required to overcome the natural resistance to flow and ensure perfusion of all body tissues. We can measure the perfusion pressure generated by the circulatory system in the form of arterial blood pressure.

Most of this perfusion pressure is generated by the pumping action of the heart and the contraction of smooth muscle in artery walls. Blood circulation is augmented by the elasticity of veins, the system of one-way valves in the blood vessels, and the contraction of skeletal muscles as you move about.

In the healthy individual, these work together to keep blood pressure relatively constant throughout a variety of activities and environmental conditions.

PROBLEM: SHOCK

Shock is the term for inadequate perfusion pressure in the circulatory system resulting in inadequate oxygenation of body cells. While even a small drop in pressure can cause poor oxygenation of tissues in the extremities and skin, compensation mechanisms will usually adjust blood flow to preserve the oxygenation and perfusion of vital organs. If pressure continues to drop, even vital body tissues will suffer. Shock is a major critical system problem requiring immediate and aggressive treatment.

Shock typically develops along a spectrum of severity from mild to severe. Progression can be stopped at any given point, but it is more common for shock to progress from bad to worse. The ability to recognize shock while there is still time to do something about it is a critical field assessment skill.

The three basic types of shock correspond to the three major components of the circulatory system. Volume shock is due to the loss of circulating blood volume. Vascular shock is caused by the loss of blood vessel muscle tone. Cardiogenic shock is caused by inadequate pumping action of the heart (i.e., poor cardiac output). In addition, acute stress reaction (ASR) can mimic some of the symptoms of shock while having none of the dangers of shock.

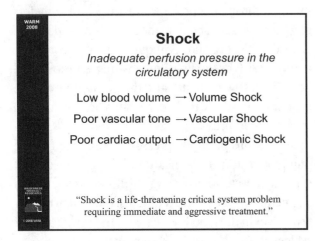

Shock

Inadequate perfusion pressure in the circulatory system

Low blood volume → Volume Shock

Poor vascular tone → Vascular Shock

Poor cardiac output → Cardiogenic Shock

"Shock is a life-threatening critical system problem requiring immediate and aggressive treatment."

VOLUME SHOCK

A history of trauma sufficient to cause severe internal or external bleeding should make you think immediately of volume shock. A more common mechanism in the wilderness environment is dehydration from diarrhea, vomiting, or sweating. Regardless of the mechanism, the problem is the same: inadequate perfusion pressure due to low blood volume.

Severe bleeding from an artery is usually easy to spot. But in some cases the fluid loss may not be so obvious. Watching the body compensate may be the only way to detect the onset of volume shock from slow internal bleeding or dehydration. We observe compensation by measuring vital signs.

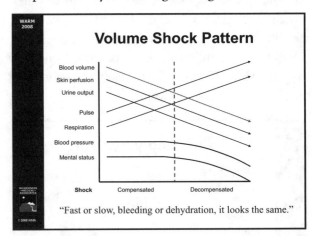

Volume Shock Pattern

"Fast or slow, bleeding or dehydration, it looks the same."

The first vital sign change to occur as shock develops is often the shell/core effect indicated by reduced skin perfusion, followed by an increase in pulse and respiratory rate. This accounts for the classic symptoms of shock described as cool pale skin and rapid pulse and rapid breathing. Dizziness may occur with standing or sitting up as brain perfusion is temporarily impaired because the circulatory system is unable to compensate for the effects of gravity.

Early on, perfusion is maintained to the vital organs of the body core through a combination of increased cardiac output, shell/core effect, and fluid shift into the blood from body cells and tissues. The rate and depth of respiration will increase to oxygenate the blood as it passes more quickly through the respiratory system.

If you are able to measure blood pressure, you may observe that the compensatory mechanisms keep it near normal in the very early stages of volume loss. Because the brain is still enjoying near-normal perfusion, the patient may exhibit only mild mental status changes. This stage is called compensated volume shock.

This serves to remind us that a single measurement of blood pressure alone is not particularly useful. It offers only an approximation of perfusion pressure at one place on the upper arm or leg. It does not reliably indicate low blood volume or the status of cellular oxygenation. Unless you are alert to the entire vital sign pattern for volume shock, you may miss the diagnosis until it is too late.

In the long-term care situation, monitoring urine output is good way to monitor the status of the circulatory system. Reduced blood volume will result in greatly reduced urine output as the kidneys do their part to conserve fluid. The urine that is produced will be more concentrated and appear dark yellow or brown. These are important signs to watch for when you're concerned about the slow loss of fluid with burns, vomiting and diarrhea, and other forms of dehydration.

As volume shock progresses and the compensation mechanisms are overwhelmed, oxygenation and perfusion of the brain will be reduced and the evolutionary onion will really start to peel. As perfusion pressure falls, level of consciousness will decrease and the brain's ability to control the circulatory and respiratory systems will become impaired. Cardiac output will decrease as heart muscle is deprived of oxygen. Circulatory collapse and respiratory failure are imminent. This is sometimes called profound or decompensated shock.

The rate of progression of volume shock will be directly related to the rate of fluid loss, but the pattern of vital sign change will be the same. In the case of severe bleeding, the patient may progress from compensated volume shock to decompensated shock within minutes. Dehydration, on the other hand, can progress over many hours or days. Either way, if volume shock cannot be reversed, the patient will die.

FIELD TREATMENT OF VOLUME SHOCK

Stop the Fluid Loss – Severe bleeding is a critical system problem identified during the initial assessment and treated as part of basic life support (Chapter 8). Dehydration is a more common mechanism for volume shock in the wilderness or offshore setting. It is less urgent but no less important, and is also initially treated by stopping the fluid loss. You will need to reduce heat stress to reduce sweating or use medication to stop diarrhea or vomiting. This may or may not be easy to accomplish depending on the situation.

Restore Blood Volume – The first aid treatments of reassurance, elevating the feet, and keeping the patient warm does nothing to address the real problem of low blood volume. A patient in volume shock from blood loss needs a surgeon and a hospital. Intravenous therapy with normal saline or other crystalloid solution is only a temporary treatment that may buy time, or possibly cause harm.

With volume shock from slow dehydration due to sweating or diarrhea, field treatment may be definitive. Intravenous fluid replacement is ideal, but oral replacement with electrolyte solution or food and water can work almost as well.

The return of normal vital signs, along with normal urine output, is the best indication of success. If the patient is not improving within a reasonable period of time, evacuation must be considered. Shock that you cannot reverse in the field is a life-threatening medical emergency regardless of its cause.

Position and Protection – Regardless of the cause of volume shock, it is important to protect the patient from heat loss. The patient in shock will not be generating much heat through metabolism or muscle activity, and hypothermia will greatly reduce the chances of survival. Contact with the ground, water, or cold IV solutions and bottled oxygen will exacerbate the problem. Be sure to add heat to the patient package in all but the warmest of conditions.

A patient in shock should be carried horizontally because the vertical orientation can inhibit perfusion of the brain and can be fatal. Avoid a vertical hoist into a helicopter or onto a ship, or a technical evacuation with the litter belayed in the vertical position.

Oxygen – Supplemental oxygen may be brought to the scene by rescue teams. Adding more oxygen to the air the patient is breathing increases the efficiency of a limited blood supply. In an emergency situation, oxygen is never harmful.

VASCULAR SHOCK

With loss of muscle tone in the arteries or the inflammation and dilation of capillaries due to injury or illness (vasodilation), the pressure exerted on the blood volume drops. The pattern of vital sign change will include an increase in pulse and respiratory rate, and a reduction in urine output. However, you may not see shell/core compensation as you do in volume shock because the blood vessels in the skin may be unable to constrict normally. This is where the appearance of vascular shock can differ from that of volume shock.

Vascular shock is most often seen in the severe, systemic allergic reaction called anaphylaxis. It can also be part of a syndrome caused by systemic infection (sepsis) or due to the loss of nervous system control in severe spinal cord injury. The result is the same: inadequate perfusion pressure in the circulatory system resulting in inadequate cellular oxygenation.

FIELD TREATMENT OF VASCULAR SHOCK

First, keep the patient horizontal because the ability to compensate for the effects of gravity is impaired. Next, treat the cause if possible. Anaphylaxis can be reversed with medication (Chapter 9). If vasodilatation is not reversible with field treatment, as in spinal cord injury or infection, evacuation and IV fluid to expand blood volume is indicated. As with volume shock, hypothermia is an anticipated problem in the wilderness setting.

CARDIOGENIC SHOCK

Cardiogenic shock results in reduced cardiac output. Reduced cardiac output is most often caused by myocardial infarction or cardiac dysrhythm (abnormal heart rhythm). We commonly call this a heart attack, well recognized as a major problem. Symptoms include chest pain or pressure, possibly accompanied by the signs and symptoms of shock. The pattern of compensation will resemble that of volume shock, except that the heart rate may be variable.

The symptoms of a heart attack may be very severe or quite subtle. Heart attack with the anticipated problem of cardiogenic shock should be on your problem list whenever a patient complains of chest discomfort without an obvious mechanism of injury. This is especially true when the patient's history includes several risk factors for coronary artery disease like smoking, obesity, hypertension, or diabetes.

Cardiogenic shock from trauma is rare. It generally occurs when blood or fluid accumulates in the pericardial sack around the heart, inhibiting heart filling and reducing cardiac output. It can also develop as a result of poor function in a contused heart. It should be suspected or anticipated whenever a trauma patient complaints of persistent chest pain. Cardiogenic shock from trauma is as serious a problem as a heart attack.

FIELD TREATMENT OF CARDIOGENIC SHOCK

Field treatment options are limited; the patient needs a hospital. Suspected myocardial ischemia is treated with oxygen, aspirin, and the patient's own nitroglycerin if the drug has been prescribed. Even ALS treatment is very temporary. This is covered in more detail in Chapter 28.

Cardiac trauma requires urgent evacuation to surgical care. ALS field treatment is limited to pericardiocentesis, which is the aspiration of excess blood or fluid from the pericardial sack. Definitive care may require cardiovascular surgery. This should be taken into account in planning your evacuation route and destination.

ACUTE STRESS REACTION (ASR)

Acute stress reaction (ASR) is the term for the frequent and normal response to emotional stress caused by fear, disappointment, surprise, pain, grief, or any number of other influences. Some texts use the term *psychogenic shock* for this phenomenon. However, while ASR can look like shock, it has none of the serious consequences.

The sympathetic form of ASR is the "speed up" response you feel when you're anxious or scared, produced by the release of the hormones epinephrine and norepinephrine. It speeds up the pulse and respiratory rate, shunts blood to the muscles, dilates the pupils, and generally gets the body ready for action. It also stimulates the release of natural hormones that serve to mask the pain of injury.

This type of ASR certainly has value to human survival. It allows extraordinary efforts even in the presence of severe injury. Unfortunately, it also makes

---

WARM 2008

ASR

Sympathetic:
- Mediated by epinephrine
- Increases pulse, respiration; reduces skin perfusion; increases anxiety
- Can look like shock or respiratory distress

Parasympathetic:
- Multiple chemical mediators
- Slows pulse, causes fainting
- Can look like TBI or other mechanism for mental status changes

WILDERNESS MEDICAL ASSOCIATES

©2008 WMA

---

the accurate assessment of injuries difficult for the rescuer by hiding pain and altering vital signs. The elevation in pulse and respiratory rate and change in mental status can mimic the volume shock pattern.

The parasympathetic form of ASR is the faint and nauseous feeling some people experience with pain or the sight of blood. Its effect slows the heart rate enough to cause a temporary loss of perfusion to the brain. The evolutionary value of this response is more difficult to figure out. This, too, is harmless except in

its ability to mimic the shell/core compensation seen in true volume shock or the change in mental status seen in brain injury.

The key to recognizing acute stress reaction is in the mechanism of injury and the progression of symptoms. ASR can look like shock but can occur with or without any mechanism of injury to cause shock. We have all seen people with only minor extremity sprains or superficial wounds become lightheaded, pale, and nauseous. Although they look shocky, there is no cause for alarm. They have no mechanism for significant volume loss.

It is important to remember that acute stress reaction can co-exist with shock. In cases where the patient has both a mechanism of injury for true shock and the signs and symptoms to go with it, you must treat it as such. With time ASR will improve; shock will not.

FIELD TREATMENT OF ASR

Allowing the patient to lie down, providing calm reassurance, and relieving pain should result in immediate improvement in symptoms. Note that this is the traditional treatment for shock described in many first aid texts. In the ambulance setting, the difference between ASR and shock is less important because both are managed as shock during the short period of treatment and transport. For long-term management in the remote setting, recognizing ASR for what it is can save a lot of resources and risk, not to mention your peace of mind.

WILDERNESS CONSIDERATIONS FOR SHOCK

The most common mechanism for volume shock in the backcountry setting is dehydration. For vascular shock, the most common is anaphylaxis. And for cardiogenic shock, it is the same as in the urban context—heart attack.

The ideal treatment for all shock is evacuation to definitive medical care. In the wilderness or offshore setting where evacuation may be impossible or involve a high level of risk, field treatment may be prolonged. In some cases like dehydration or anaphylaxis, the field treatment may be definitive.

Your worry list includes situations where you cannot reverse the progression of shock and signs and symptoms that indicate a poor response to treatment. These cases may be worth a high-risk evacuation or an attempt to bring advanced level care to the patient. The balance of risk versus benefit will depend on the situation and the experience and skill of the practitioner making the judgment.

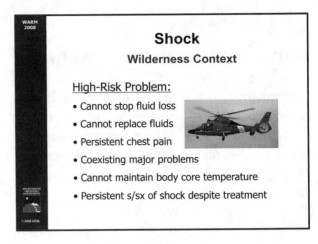

Shock
Wilderness Context

High-Risk Problem:
- Cannot stop fluid loss
- Cannot replace fluids
- Persistent chest pain
- Coexisting major problems
- Cannot maintain body core temperature
- Persistent s/sx of shock despite treatment

NOTES:

The Respiratory System

5

STRUCTURE AND FUNCTION

The respiratory system brings air into close contact with the circulating blood to allow for the exchange of oxygen and carbon dioxide. The de-oxygenated blood returning from the body enters the right side of the heart. Contraction of the right ventricle pumps it into the pulmonary circulation where the capillary beds in the lungs surround millions of alveolar air sacks, providing a blood-to-air interface the size of a tennis court.

The gas exchange takes place in these alveoli, where only a thin semi-permeable membrane separates air from blood. Oxygen is actively transported across the alveolar membrane to bind with hemoglobin in red blood cells. Carbon dioxide diffuses passively from the blood plasma across the membrane into the air to be exhaled. The oxygenated blood then returns via the pulmonary veins to the heart, where the strong muscle of the left ventricle recirculates it to body tissues.

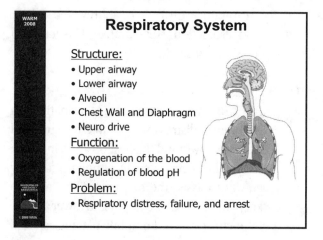

Respiratory System

Structure:
• Upper airway
• Lower airway
• Alveoli
• Chest Wall and Diaphragm
• Neuro drive

Function:
• Oxygenation of the blood
• Regulation of blood pH

Problem:
• Respiratory distress, failure, and arrest

The efficiency with which the system works is measured as oxygen saturation. A healthy person at sea level would measure 98–100% on a pulse oximeter, indicating that the oxygen carrying capacity of the blood is completely filled. At high altitude or in the presence of respiratory problems, oxygen saturation will fall, indicating less efficient respiration. It is also easy to measure the efficiency of the respiratory system by assessing mental status and skin color.

Like the circulatory system, the structure of the respiratory system can be described in basic terms for field use: upper airway, lower airway, alveoli, chest wall and diaphragm, and nervous system control. The upper and lower airways consist of the semi-rigid tubes that conduct air into the alveoli. These passages are lined with mucous membrane designed to continuously remove contaminants and bacteria from the system. The upward flow of mucous is generated by tiny hair-like structures called *cilia*. You are continuously swallowing the resulting mixture, usually without thinking about it.

The chest wall and diaphragm create a bellows system that draws the air in and out. The rate and depth of breathing is under nervous system control. In a healthy patient, the brain regulates breathing by measuring the pH (acidity) of the blood. This is actually a reflection of the amount of carbon dioxide dissolved in the blood plasma. Too much carbon dioxide in the blood causes an increase in acidity. The brain responds by increasing the rate and depth of respiration to "blow off" the carbon dioxide until normal acidity is reestablished. Conversely, alkalosis (decreased acidity) is corrected by decreasing the rate and depth of respiration to retain carbon dioxide.

This acid/base regulation system is very precise and results in a smooth and regular respiratory pattern. But in some disease conditions like emphysema, the amount of carbon dioxide in the blood is high all the time because the lower airway is chronically constricted and cannot ventilate properly. The brain then falls back on measuring the amount of oxygen in the blood to determine breathing rate and depth.

This is much less precise, is more easily upset, and results in a more irregular pattern.

RESPIRATORY PROBLEMS

Respiratory distress is the generic term for difficulty breathing. Symptoms include increased respiratory rate, increased respiratory effort, anxiety, and noise like wheezing and coughing. One of the most obvious signs of respiratory distress is the use of accessory muscles.

Normally, a person at rest uses only the diaphragm to breathe. When work is increased, oxygen demand increases and the respiratory system will use muscles in the chest, shoulders, and neck to increase the depth of respiration. You would expect to see this as a normal response in someone who is running or hiking hard. You would not expect to see it in someone sitting still. Accessory muscle use at rest indicates respiratory distress.

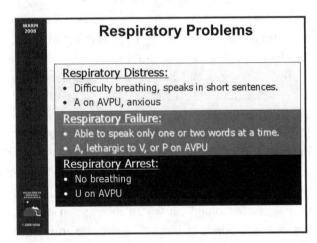

A more subtle sign is shortness of breath on exertion. This patient has a compromised respiratory system that is only capable of supplying enough oxygen if the demand is low. Sitting and resting is fine but any level of increased exertion, like hiking, causes severe shortness of breath. This symptom is often an early sign of respiratory distress due to pneumonia, high altitude pulmonary edema, or asthma.

Whatever the cause of respiratory distress, it will eventually progress to respiratory failure if not corrected. Respiratory failure means that the system cannot supply enough oxygen to the blood to keep the brain functioning normally. The primary indicator is decay in mental status and level of consciousness in the presence of difficulty breathing. If not corrected, the inevitable result will be respiratory arrest.

Another sign of respiratory failure is the inability to speak more than a few words between breaths. This is called *one- or two-word dyspnea*. To illustrate what this looks like, imagine trying to speak easily after sprinting hard for 500 meters or so. A patient in this condition at rest is in serious trouble. Conversely, a patient who is able to talk at length about their shortness of breath is probably okay for now.

Respiratory distress that you cannot fix in the field is a major problem with this critical body system. The progression to failure may be rapid or slow. The treatment and evacuation may be a desperate emergency or a careful and low-stress process depending on the rate of progression.

GENERIC TREATMENT FOR RESPIRATORY DISTRESS

Respiratory distress is one of the most frightening problems that you will ever deal with in emergency medicine. Your immediate response should be to get treatment going while you develop a more specific assessment and plan. The generic treatment for all forms of respiratory distress is abbreviated PROP: Position and Protection, Reassurance, Oxygen, and Positive Pressure Ventilation.

PROP

Position and Protection: Any patient in respiratory distress who is able to move will have already found the best position in which to breathe. This is usually sitting up to allow gravity to assist the diaphragm and to help keep fluids out of the upper and lower airway. In unconscious or immobile patients, special care must be taken to position them in a way that protects the airway from obstruction or aspiration of vomit, blood, and secretions.

Reassurance: Encourage the patient to breathe slower and deeper, rather than panting like a dog. This brings in fresh oxygen rather than moving the same old carbon dioxide back and forth in the airways.

Oxygen: If available, giving supplemental oxygen from a tank or concentrator may increase the amount of oxygen getting into the blood, and ultimately to the brain.

Positive Pressure Ventilation: A patient in respiratory distress will fatigue rapidly. You may need to provide positive pressure ventilation to assist the patient's efforts. You do not need to wait until the patient goes into respiratory arrest to use this technique.

SPECIFIC TREATMENTS FOR RESPIRATORY DISTRESS

Beyond PROP, more specific treatment for respiratory distress will depend on which part of the respiratory system is affected. Although PROP may significantly improve symptoms in some cases, it may be nearly ineffective in others. Being able to identify the specific type of respiratory system problem during your initial assessment, focused history, and physical exam will allow for a more effective and focused treatment.

UPPER AIRWAY OBSTRUCTION

The upper airway can be obstructed by the tongue, a piece of food, or swelling from trauma or infection. The obstruction may be partial or complete. With partial obstruction, the patient will have noisy and labored respiration characterized by wheezing, whistling, or stridor—the high-pitched raspy sound made by inhalation against an obstruction. The ability to swallow saliva may be impaired, causing the patient to drool. Talking may be difficult or impossible.

With a partial obstruction, the first rule of treatment is, "Do no harm". Any attempt to remove

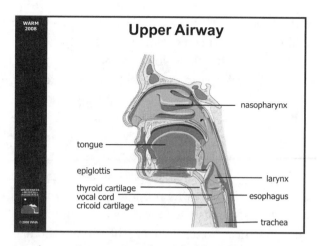

an obstruction carries the risk of making it worse. If the patient is not yet in respiratory failure, the ideal treatment is urgent evacuation to advanced life support and surgical care.

When the patient is in respiratory failure or arrest, immediate basic life support techniques are used to clear the airway (Chapter 8). At this point, the benefit is lifesaving and you have nothing to lose by trying. In cases where a foreign object is removed before the patient gets in real trouble, you may certainly take credit for the save. Remember, though, that the object may have caused enough irritation to create the anticipated problem of swelling, which can lead to further obstruction later on. Evacuation would be prudent if the insult was severe, such as a burn from hot food.

Airway obstruction due to swelling from burns, trauma, or infection is the most difficult to manage in the field. A partial obstruction carries the anticipated problem of complete obstruction, which can develop quickly in some cases. The patient will naturally find the best airway position, and there is little else you can do to improve on it. Airway obstruction due to swelling is best evacuated urgently to advanced life support and surgical care.

LOWER AIRWAY CONSTRICTION

Spasm, swelling of the mucous membrane lining, or the accumulation of mucous or pus can cause narrowing of the bronchi and bronchioles, which are the tubes of the lower airway. This is what happens in asthma, bronchitis, and anaphylaxis. The constriction inhibits the movement of air in and out of the alveoli. In the initial stages of lower airway constriction, the patient may have a more difficult time exhaling than inhaling. This can render positive pressure ventilation less effective, although the rest of the generic treatment for respiratory distress is certainly useful.

In severe constriction, inspiration and expiration are often prolonged with pronounced wheezing and a cough. Sometimes the lower airway noise is loud enough to hear from a distance. Other times you may need a stethoscope or an ear to the patient's chest.

The most frequent cause of life-threatening lower airway constriction is asthma (Chapter 10). In the absence of a clear history, look for an exposure to smoke, inhaled water, or other irritating substance. Look for hives, facial swelling, and a history of allergic exposure that may indicate the severe allergic reaction called anaphylaxis. There may be a history of slowly

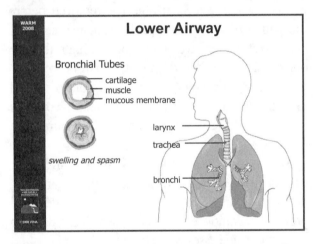

Lower Airway

Bronchial Tubes
cartilage
muscle
mucous membrane

swelling and spasm

larynx
trachea
bronchi

worsening illness and fever pointing to respiratory infection. There may be an obvious increase in respiratory effort as the system struggles to move air against increased resistance. The vital sign pattern will reveal the compensatory mechanisms in the form of elevated heart and respiratory rate.

Lower airway constriction as a result of asthma, anaphylaxis, or any other mechanism is a major problem when it causes respiratory distress. Your initial response should PROP; the ideal treatment is medication to relieve the constriction and treat the cause.

Bronchodilators such as nebulized albuterol may be helpful in cases of bronchitis or smoke inhalation. Antibiotics may be added for infection. With a history of asthma or anaphylaxis, you can follow the Wilderness Protocols detailed in chapters 9 and 10.

FLUID IN THE ALVEOLI

Excess fluid accumulates in the alveoli blocking the exchange of oxygen and carbon dioxide between air and blood. The source is usually capillary leakage within the lung as part of an inflammatory process caused by infection or inhalation injury. Contusion of lung tissue can result in pulmonary edema. This should be an anticipated problem with suspected rib fracture or any blow to the chest severe enough to "knock the wind out of you." Capillary leakage can also be the result of congestive heart failure or the effect of reduced oxygen at high altitude. Contusion or laceration of the lung tissue may cause the alveoli to fill with blood.

Shortness of breath on exertion will reveal the reduced lung capacity in the early stages of fluid accumulation. The patient often develops a dry cough as the lung tries to clear itself. A low-grade fever may develop. In the presence of a mechanism of injury like submersion, high altitude pulmonary edema, chest trauma, or infection, these early signs are reason to anticipate respiratory distress as the situation becomes worse.

As the problem progresses, small amounts of fluid

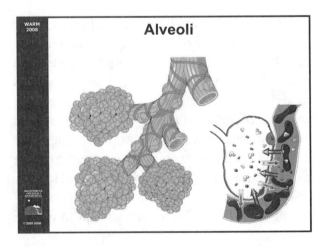

Alveoli

may be heard with a stethoscope or an ear to the chest as the patient breathes. The sound is called rales and is roughly reproducible by sucking air through a wet sponge. Large amounts of fluid in the lungs will cause gurgling that can be heard at a distance. Fluid may actually froth from the mouth and may be tinged with pus or blood. At this point, respiratory distress will have become obvious, with imminent respiratory failure.

With alveolar fluid, PROP can make a significant difference. Positive pressure ventilation can help force alveolar fluid back into the circulatory system restoring lung surface area for gas exchange. You don't have to wait for the patient to stop breathing to apply PPV. This is a safe and effective basic life support treatment for respiratory distress. Don't worry about timing; a patient in trouble will adjust his respiratory effort to your efforts to assist.

The patient will prefer to sit up, even on a litter during evacuation. Supplemental oxygen will help and should be an early part of the plan for treatment and evacuation. Definitive care will require antibiotics for infection or medication to reduce edema from other causes. Access to advanced life support is high priority. For high altitude pulmonary edema, the definitive treatment is immediate descent, but there are medications that can buy the patient some time (Chapter 18).

CHEST WALL TRAUMA

Trauma to the chest wall or diaphragm can interfere with the function of the respiratory system in a number of ways, but the most common is pain from a fractured rib. The effective application of PROP and pain relief will often significantly improve the respiratory status of the trauma patient. Sometimes a rib belt or wrap around the chest will make the patient more comfortable and improve respiratory effort. If you choose to apply a belt, monitor the patient carefully and be prepared to remove it if the belt seems to make matters worse.

More serious structural damage to the chest wall or pain that does not respond quickly to field treatment deserves urgent evacuation. An unstable chest wall, also called a flail chest, indicates that the bellows system is damaged to the point that it is no longer rigid. Instead of the lungs expanding with inspiration, the chest wall collapses. Hemothorax and pneumothorax are terms used to describe the presence of blood and/or air in the chest cavity in the space between the lungs and the chest wall. This prevents full expansion of the lungs, shifts the heart and airways out of position, and puts pressure on the great vessels of the circulatory system. In the rare case of an open pneumothorax, sometimes called a sucking chest wound, air may enter the chest cavity through a hole in the chest wall. The usual cause is a knife or gunshot wound.

Signs of pneumothorax include hyperexpansion of the chest, deviation of the trachea to one side, and reduced pulse pressure. There may be bruising, fractured ribs, or other direct evidence of injury. Bleeding within the chest may result in volume shock with the associated pattern of vital sign changes.

The generic treatment for respiratory distress, like the field treatment for volume shock, is limited

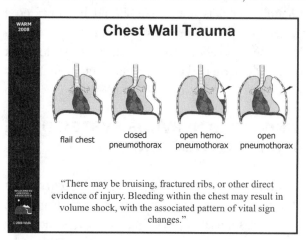

Chest Wall Trauma

flail chest | closed pneumothorax | open hemo-pneumothorax | open pneumothorax

"There may be bruising, fractured ribs, or other direct evidence of injury. Bleeding within the chest may result in volume shock, with the associated pattern of vital sign changes."

and temporary only. The patient with chest injury significant enough to cause respiratory distress deserves immediate evacuation. Assist the patient into whatever position allows for the best respiration and the least pain.

Open chest wounds with air bubbling in and out of the defect should be covered with an air tight seal, like a piece of plastic bag or duct tape. You do not need to make a one-way valve or coordinate the patch placement with inspiration. Just put it on. If applying a patch improves the situation, leave it in place. If symptoms become worse, remove it.

DECREASED NERVOUS SYSTEM DRIVE (HYPOVENTILATION)

Breathing is controlled by the brain. If the brain is not functioning correctly, breathing may be irregular or slow. If the brain stops working, breathing will stop. The possible causes include problems like low blood sugar, hypothermia, and toxins.

The symptoms present in marked contrast to the other forms of respiratory distress. Decreased nervous system drive is not noisy or fast. Because the patient's level of consciousness is already reduced by the primary nervous system problem, mental status it is no longer a reliable indicator of brain oxygenation. The patient is not awake enough to tell you that she is having trouble breathing. You won't see it unless you look for it!

Any injured or ill person with slow or irregular breathing who is not awake should be considered in need of positive pressure ventilation and oxygen. Don't be timid about this. PPV carries a very low risk of causing harm and great benefit if the patient really needs it.

INCREASED NERVOUS SYSTEM DRIVE (HYPERVENTILATION)

Increased nervous system drive occurs with altitude, exercise, injury, and illness. This is a normal response to physiologic demands requiring more oxygen and producing more carbon dioxide. Increased respiration also occurs with acute stress reaction, but not in response to an increased need.

The result of hyperventilation in ASR can be to abnormally decrease the carbon dioxide concentration in the blood with the associated abnormal increase in pH. This is blood chemistry out of balance that can produce a variety of nervous system symptoms that are referred to as *hyperventilation syndrome*.

Typically, the patient will complain of tingling of the hands and feet, and numbness around the mouth. The patient may feel paralyzed but his ability to move is not actually impaired. Vision may be affected with the patient seeing spots or a narrowed visual field. The symptoms may fuel further ASR that exacerbates the hyperventilation. The patient may ultimately faint, which will cure the hyperventilation.

Hyperventilation can occur with or without obvious fast and heavy breathing. It only takes a slight increase in depth and rate over time to cause changes in blood chemistry. The respiratory changes observed in your measurement of vital signs may be very subtle. Fortunately, the condition is self-limiting.

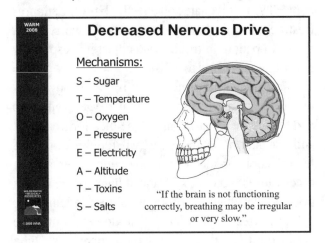

WARM 2008

Decreased Nervous Drive

Mechanisms:

S – Sugar
T – Temperature
O – Oxygen
P – Pressure
E – Electricity
A – Altitude
T – Toxins
S – Salts

"If the brain is not functioning correctly, breathing may be irregular or very slow."

It can be difficult to distinguish between hyperventilation syndrome and major critical system problems, especially if there is a positive mechanism for injury. As with other components of acute stress reaction, however, it gets better with time, pain management and relief of anxiety. Reassuring the patient that hyperventilation is the cause of their symptoms almost always cures it. Coach the patient to breathe slower.

WILDERNESS CONSIDERATIONS FOR RESPIRATORY DISTRESS

As with shock, the ideal treatment for respiratory distress is evacuation to definitive medical care. In the wilderness or offshore setting where evacuation may be impossible or involve a high level of risk, field treatment may be prolonged. In some cases like asthma, anaphylaxis, or airway obstruction, field treatment may be definitive.

Your worry list includes situations where you cannot reverse the progression of respiratory distress or signs and symptoms that indicate a poor response to treatment. These cases may be worth a high-risk evacuation or an attempt to bring advanced level care to the patient. The balance of risk versus benefit will depend on the situation and the experience and skill of the practitioner making the judgment.

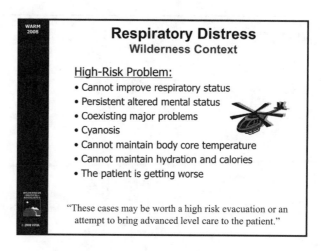

Respiratory Distress
Wilderness Context

<u>High-Risk Problem:</u>
• Cannot improve respiratory status
• Persistent altered mental status
• Coexisting major problems
• Cyanosis
• Cannot maintain body core temperature
• Cannot maintain hydration and calories
• The patient is getting worse

"These cases may be worth a high risk evacuation or an attempt to bring advanced level care to the patient."

NOTES:

NOTES:

The Central Nervous System

STRUCTURE AND FUNCTION

The central nervous system controls all critical life functions, both voluntary and involuntary. The brain receives stimuli directly from the eyes, nose, and facial nerves via the cranial nerves in the head, and indirectly from the rest of the body through peripheral nerves and spinal cord.

The soft tissue of the brain and spinal cord are well protected within the bony structure of the skull and vertebrae of the spine. From the gap between the individual vertebrae, unprotected peripheral nerves branch out from the spinal cord to reach all body tissues. Nerves controlling the most critical functions of the major body systems exit the cord at the base of the skull and the upper part of the cervical spine. A number of problems, often serious, can affect the central nervous system.

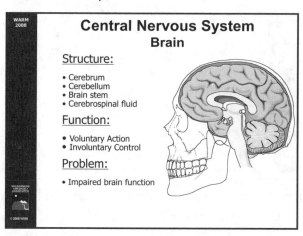

IMPAIRED BRAIN FUNCTION

Because nervous system tissue is exquisitely sensitive to oxygen deprivation, any significant problem with oxygenation and perfusion will affect mental status. A subtle change in brain function is often the first indication of a serious condition. This is the peeling of the evolutionary onion.

For field purposes, we describe brain function by using a scale abbreviated AVPU. This simple assessment tool is familiar to most emergency care providers. More complex evaluation tools, such as the Glasgow Coma Scale, are generally not as useful for wilderness medicine.

AVPU Scale
A - Awake: Refined by describing Mental Status (M/S).
V - Verbal: Responds to verbal stimuli.
P - Pain: Responds only to painful stimuli.
U - Unresponsive.

In the Emergency Medical Services, normal mental status in the awake patient is often abbreviated A&O x 4. This means that the patient is awake and oriented to person, place, time, and event. Using this phrase to describe normal mental status is fine as long as everyone knows what you're talking about. This description becomes confusing when the patient is not normal. Reporting a patient as "A&O x 2" gives little useful information.

In describing mental status, plain language is usually better in wilderness or disaster settings that may involve multiple agencies and medical personnel at various levels of training. By describing your patient as "awake, knows her name and where she is, but not sure how she got here or what day of the week is," may seem cumbersome, but everyone involved in her care and transport will understand it. Furthermore, improvement or decay in mental status will be more easily detected.

DIFFERENTIAL DIAGNOSIS OF IMPAIRED BRAIN FUNCTION

The differential diagnosis is a list of the possible causes of a condition or problem. The most common causes of impaired brain function can be summarized as a simple differential diagnosis with the acronym STOPEATS.

STOPEATS

S - Sugar: blood sugar, low or high

T - Temperature: hypothermia or hyperthermia

O - Oxygen: hypoxia from suffocation or drowning

P - Pressure: increased intracranial pressure, or decreased perfusion pressure.

E - Electricity: manmade current or lightning

A - Altitude: hypoxia from HAPE, pressure from HACE

T - Toxins: ingested, inhaled, injected, or surface absorbed

S - Salts: electrolyte imbalance such as exertional hyponatremia

STOPEATS can be a handy diagnostic tool when you are evaluating mental status changes in the presence of a mixed or uncertain mechanism of injury. While reviewing the mnemonic, you will usually be able to eliminate some possible causes in your survey of the scene and examination of the patient. Other possibilities will have to remain on your problem list until they can be ruled out or confirmed over time.

Imagine caring for the subject of a successful 48-hour backcountry search. Your patient is found curled up under a spruce tree in a level area of forest at 950 meters in elevation. The weather is cool and wet without thunderstorm activity. He is V on the APVU scale and shivering. There is no evidence of trauma.

Already, you can eliminate problems with pressure, electricity, oxygen, and altitude from your problem list. Even though you are fairly certain that his problem is hypothermia, the mnemonic reminds you to consider

blood sugar, toxins, and salts as possible contributing factors. Time and response to treatment may allow you to further refine your problem list in the field, or you may have to keep a potential problem on the list throughout an evacuation effort. This is the Big Net principle at work. Treat what you can, and evacuate for what you can't.

INCREASED INTRACRANIAL PRESSURE (ICP)

This is the P in the STOPEATS mnemonic, and the brain problem that is most likely to be fatal. Like other body tissues, the brain will swell when injured. Unlike other tissues, the brain is confined within the rigid structure of the cranium. Bleeding or the development of edema within this limited space can produce a rise in intracranial pressure that inhibits perfusion of brain tissue. Causes include traumatic brain injury, high altitude cerebral edema (HACE), and brain damage due to hypoxia. Stroke and

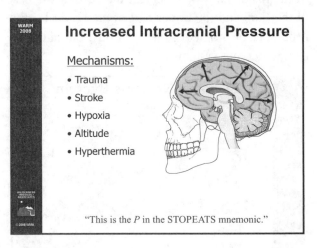

Increased Intracranial Pressure

Mechanisms:
- Trauma
- Stroke
- Hypoxia
- Altitude
- Hyperthermia

"This is the *P* in the STOPEATS mnemonic."

hyperthermia are less common, but can also lead to swelling and increased intracranial pressure.

Like shock, increased ICP has a typical pattern and spectrum of severity regardless of its cause or rate of onset. Although other vital sign changes occur, altered mental status ("peeling the onion") is often the earliest vital sign indicator of increasing ICP. The patient may be disoriented or appear intoxicated, combative, or restless. These signs will typically be accompanied by severe headache, photophobia (discomfort with bright light), and nausea. If the pressure continues to increase, the deeper layers of brain function will begin to show the effects with the onset of vomiting, adding the anticipated problems of airway obstruction and dehydration.

Symptoms of severe increased ICP include a decrease in the level of consciousness with seizures, posturing, and pupil dilation as the brain stem is pressed through the floor of the cranium. At this point, survival without neurosurgical intervention is unlikely. In the ideal situation, any patient with increased ICP as an anticipated problem is evacuated from the field before it develops.

FIELD TREATMENT OF INCREASED ICP

The rapid onset of increased ICP from severe intracranial bleeding will be fatal in most backcountry or offshore situations. Cardiopulmonary arrest due to severe brain damage does not respond to CPR or defibrillation. It is the early recognition of slow-onset swelling from the accumulation of edema fluid that can save lives. The appropriate response is good basic life support and urgent evacuation.

There is no field treatment specific to increased ICP that will improve survival. However, your careful attention to basic life support including airway control, ventilation, preservation of body core temperature, and hydration can certainly improve the outcome. Evacuation to surgical care is a priority, but support of vital body functions during the evacuation is equally essential.

TRAUMATIC BRAIN INJURY (TBI)

Traumatic brain injury (TBI) is the common term for brain damage from trauma. The term head injury is also commonly used, but can be confused with injuries to the face or soft tissue that may not include brain injury. TBI is diagnosed in the field by observing or obtaining a history of a change in brain function at the time of injury. The change may be as dramatic as a ten minute loss of consciousness, or as

subtle as a brief loss of memory or short period of disorientation.

Any traumatic brain injury carries the anticipated problem (A') of increased ICP. Generally, the more severe the injury, the more likely the brain is to swell. A very brief loss of consciousness or a loss of memory for the event only would suggest mild injury. Severe injury is evidenced by profound and prolonged changes in mental status, loss of memory

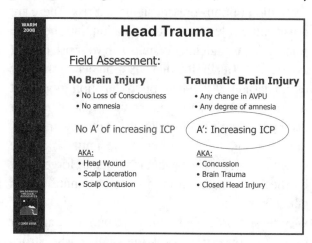

for the hours before the event, or persistent lapses of memory after the event.

Being able to diagnose TBI in the field is as advantageous as being able to determine when a patient does not have one. Injuries to the face and scalp without a change in brain function do not carry the anticipated problem of increased ICP. There may be an ugly scalp laceration or a broken nose, but if the patient has normal mental status and remembers everything that happened, there is no brain injury. At sea, as in the mountains, it is just as important to know when you don't have a medical emergency as when you do.

TRAUMATIC BRAIN INJURY: WILDERNESS CONTEXT

When TBI is on the problem list, the important question becomes whether the injured brain tissue will swell enough to cause a dangerous increase in ICP. This is a common backcountry medical dilemma. Evacuate now, or wait and watch? When is TBI a high-risk problem?

The answer is easy when the level of consciousness remains severely altered. Emergency evacuation is ideal. Even with minor TBI, obtaining a medical evaluation is a good idea when the risk of evacuation is minimal. Increased ICP is a major critical system problem, and its presence on your anticipated problem list, however unlikely, is of real concern.

The decision becomes more difficult when your evacuation options present significant risk. There are no absolute rules to fit every situation, but there are some general guidelines to help with your risk/benefit assessment. Generally, there is a higher probability of increasing ICP when brain function does not return to normal shortly after the event. Persistent disorientation or the inability to retain new memory (a condition known as anterograde amnesia) can be an ominous sign. The patient may literally forget what has been happening from minute to minute as you talk to him.

Amnesia for a significant time period is another cause for concern. This is the climber who struck his head and now doesn't know where he is, how he came to be there, or with whom. He may not know the month or time of year. This indicates a more severe

idea how severe a previous brain injury might have been, ask if the patient was hospitalized.

Evidence of skull fracture tells you that your patient has sustained a significant impact. The potential for bleeding and swelling is increased. The patient is also at risk for infection.

FIELD TREATMENT OF TRAUMATIC BRAIN INJURY

In a remote setting, it is ideal evacuate a TBI patient early, rather than waiting for the condition to become worse. This is especially true of a patient with history and symptoms that suggest a high probability of increasing ICP. You must consider the possibility of spine injury, which has the same mechanism as a TBI. Spine assessment and treatment is discussed in detail in Chapter 7.

Beyond basic life support and careful monitoring, there is no specific field treatment for TBI. If you choose to keep the patient in the field, it is important to monitor him carefully for at least 24 hours to detect the onset of brain swelling. Patients being monitored should not use narcotic or stimulant drugs or drink alcohol because this will confuse the assessment of

---

Traumatic Brain Injury
A': Increasing ICP

Field Treatment:

- Early evacuation is ideal
- Monitor 24 hours for increasing ICP
- Sleep is OK, but not alone
- Anticipate vomiting and airway obstruction
- Anticipate dehydration and hypothermia
- Pain medications (APAP preferred)
- Avoid another TBI

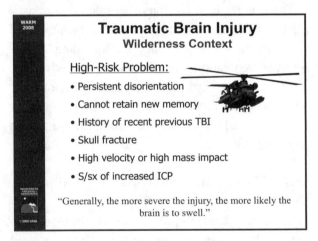

Traumatic Brain Injury
Wilderness Context

High-Risk Problem:

- Persistent disorientation
- Cannot retain new memory
- History of recent previous TBI
- Skull fracture
- High velocity or high mass impact
- S/sx of increased ICP

"Generally, the more severe the injury, the more likely the brain is to swell."

---

brain injury than the patient who may not remember the accident itself, but remembers everything else.

A history of previous TBI is also worrisome, especially if it was within the past few weeks. Incompletely healed brain tissue is prone to swelling and scar tissue is more prone to bleeding. To get an

mental status. Someone should be with the patient at all times, but it is not necessary to keep the patient awake. He will not sleep through the pain and vomiting indicative of increasing ICP.

Because vomiting is one of the signs you're watching for, you must include airway obstruction and dehydration on your anticipated problem list. The patient will not be moving around much, so he is also at risk for hypothermia in all but the warmest of environments. Basic life support in long-term care includes positioning your patient for airway control, maintaining hydration, and preserving body core temperature.

POST CONCUSSIVE SYNDROME

Following a blow to the head, some patients experience symptoms including headache, photophobia, nausea, sleep disturbance, and dizziness developing a day or so after the injury. This can occur with or without TBI. This is post concussive syndrome and rarely indicates increasing ICP. The patient may be observed and treated symptomatically.

The symptoms of post concussive syndrome can be expected to wax and wane and may persist for days or weeks. Generally, non-urgent medical follow-up is adequate. However, progressive worsening or the appearance of new symptoms such as persistent vomiting should motivate urgent evacuation and early medical evaluation.

STROKE

Stroke is the term for localized brain dysfunction caused by ischemia due to a ruptured blood vessel or the development of an obstruction in an artery. Obstruction can be caused by the formation of a clot or an embolus traveling from a distant location. The initial effect may be localized, or very extensive. Increased ICP may soon follow, especially with a stroke due to intracranial bleeding.

A sudden change in brain function without a history of trauma or intoxication should make you think of stroke. It may be as subtle as a little numbness in one hand or arm or a slight facial droop, or as dramatic as complete paralysis of one side of the body or the sudden loss of the ability to speak. In some cases, the symptoms are transient, resolving after a few minutes or hours as a clot forms and then dissolves. These transient ischemic attacks should be taken as a warning of serious and permanent problems to come if the patient is not treated soon.

TREATMENT OF STROKE

Like a heart attack, a stroke is an example of ischemia leading to infarction in a critical body system. It is a major problem, and the patient needs a hospital. During evacuation, apply basic life support and treat as you would any patient with existing or anticipated increased ICP. Do not give aspirin or ibuprofen in an effort to reduce clotting. The stroke may actually be caused by bleeding, and you will have no way of knowing that in the field.

SEIZURES

Seizure is a symptom of brain injury, not a disease unto itself. In the wilderness context, seizure may occur with low blood sugar, heat stroke, hypoxia, increased ICP, lightning injury, HACE, toxins, or hyponatremia. You will recognize this list from the STOPEATS mnemonic. The problem may be relatively mild, or very severe. Either way, the new onset of seizure activity indicates nervous system problems that may become significantly worse over time.

Of course, seizure can also be a relatively benign occurrence in a patient with a known seizure disorder such as epilepsy. The stress of backcountry travel or a voyage at sea can upset the blood levels of anti-seizure medication allowing a break-through event. This is a surprisingly common problem in the backcountry. The medical practitioner should be alert to this possibility when a seizure occurs without an obvious mechanism of injury. With organized trips or outdoors schools, it is possible that a patient with epilepsy will have chosen not to disclose this history on an intake medical form.

There are many types of seizures. The classic grand mal seizure is what you are most likely to see and is characterized by generalized tensing of all body muscles and repetitive, purposeless movement. Although the eyes may be open, the patient will be unresponsive during the seizure. He may be incontinent of feces and urine. There will usually be a period of drowsiness and disorientation after the seizure has ended.

TREATMENT OF SEIZURE

Protection from injury is the most important treatment that you can provide. Most seizures will resolve spontaneously in a short period of time. Protect the patient from injury when falling or thrashing. Also protect the patient from unnecessary treatments like chest compressions or rescuers trying to force objects between the patient's teeth.

Seizing patients will normally hold their breath briefly and become cyanotic (blue from lack of oxygenation). This is not a problem as long as it does not last more than a couple of minutes. Position the patient and ventilate if necessary after the seizure has resolved, or during the seizure if you feel that respirations are inadequate. The real worry, of course, is not the seizure itself but what may have caused it.

In the presence of a mechanism of injury like trauma or asphyxia, emergency evacuation should be initiated. In the case of a known epileptic who improves spontaneously and seems otherwise okay, evacuation need not be an emergency. However, blood levels of medication will need to be checked and adjusted. The patient should not be allowed to perform risky activities or be left alone in dangerous situations. This is not a patient who can be trusted to belay a climbing partner or remain on the deck of a small boat by himself.

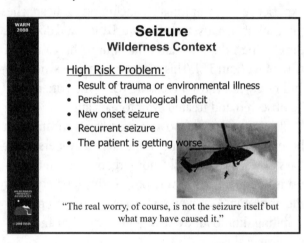

Seizure
Wilderness Context

High Risk Problem:
• Result of trauma or environmental illness
• Persistent neurological deficit
• New onset seizure
• Recurrent seizure
• The patient is getting worse

"The real worry, of course, is not the seizure itself but what may have caused it."

NOTES:

Spine Injury

7

The possibility of spine injury has long been a major concern for emergency medical personnel. The worry is that an unstable spinal column could cause or exacerbate injury to the spinal cord during extrication and transport. Structurally this seems to makes sense and stabilizing the spine in the presence of a positive mechanism of injury seems to be justified. In most EMS situations, the risk involved in

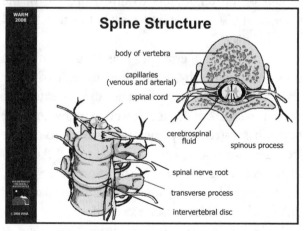

ambulance transport is minimal and the practice of stabilizing on mechanism remains protocol.

The wilderness or technical rescue setting can be considerably more challenging. Spine stabilization can substantially increase the complexity and risk

involved in care and evacuation. The wilderness medical practitioner must be able to identify those patients for whom the benefit of stabilization justifies these associated risks.

The term *positive mechanism of injury* describes any event that could cause damage to the bones, cartilage, and ligaments of the spine. A 10-meter fall onto a scree slope is obviously a positive mechanism. A stiff neck from sleeping on the cold ground is obviously not. In between, the assessment of mechanism becomes a judgment made by the practitioner based on the survey of the scene, history, and exam.

The signs and symptoms of spine injury are the same as those for other musculoskeletal trauma: pain, tenderness, swelling, deformity, dysfunction, and injury to surrounding soft tissue. In this case, the soft tissue of greatest concern is the spinal cord and peripheral nerve roots. In some cases, a patient may be unaware of a spine injury due to altered mental status, being distracted by ASR, or the pain of other trauma.

SPINE ASSESSMENT CRITERIA

Spine assessment criteria allow the rescuer to determine the need and justification for spine stabilization in the presence of an uncertain or positive mechanism of injury. This examination specifically evaluates patient reliability and looks for any history and physical exam findings consistent with spine injury. It requires a calm and cooperative patient, and a conscientious examiner. Several large-scale studies have demonstrated the effectiveness of spine assessment criteria when applied correctly.

Each element of the assessment is important. Until you are very comfortable with the concept and process, we recommend that spine evaluation be performed as

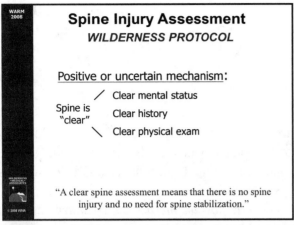

Spine Injury Assessment
WILDERNESS PROTOCOL

Positive or uncertain mechanism:

Spine is "clear"
- Clear mental status
- Clear history
- Clear physical exam

"A clear spine assessment means that there is no spine injury and no need for spine stabilization."

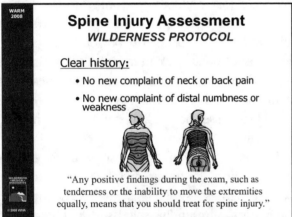

Spine Injury Assessment
WILDERNESS PROTOCOL

Clear history:
- No new complaint of neck or back pain
- No new complaint of distal numbness or weakness

"Any positive findings during the exam, such as tenderness or the inability to move the extremities equally, means that you should treat for spine injury."

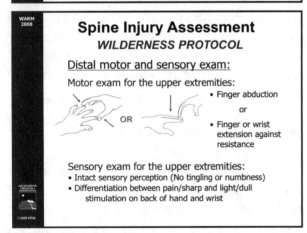

Spine Injury Assessment
WILDERNESS PROTOCOL

Distal motor and sensory exam:

Motor exam for the upper extremities:

OR

- Finger abduction

or

- Finger or wrist extension against resistance

Sensory exam for the upper extremities:
- Intact sensory perception (No tingling or numbness)
- Differentiation between pain/sharp and light/dull stimulation on back of hand and wrist

Spine Injury Assessment
WILDERNESS PROTOCOL

Clear physical exam:
- No tenderness to firm spine palpation
- Intact distal motor/sensory exam:
  - finger abduction, wrist extension
  - plantar and dorsi-flexion of feet or toes
  - sharp/dull discrimination

"On physical examination, there should be no tenderness to firm palpation of the spine, and distal motor and sensory function should be fully intact."

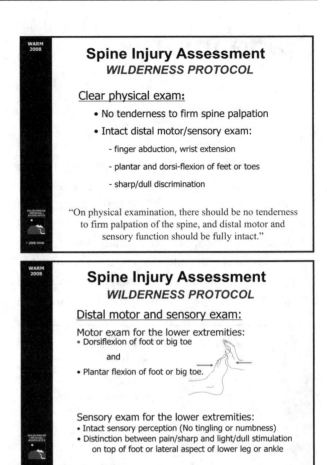

Spine Injury Assessment
WILDERNESS PROTOCOL

Distal motor and sensory exam:

Motor exam for the lower extremities:
- Dorsiflexion of foot or big toe

and

- Plantar flexion of foot or big toe.

Sensory exam for the lower extremities:
- Intact sensory perception (No tingling or numbness)
- Distinction between pain/sharp and light/dull stimulation on top of foot or lateral aspect of lower leg or ankle

a discrete process rather than incorporated into your focused history physical exam. As with any other part of your exam, spine assessment will not be reliable if the patient has altered mental status or is distracted by pain, anxiety, or other rescuers.

If you are confident that your patient is calm, cooperative, sober, and alert, your assessment can be considered reliable. To "clear" the spine, there should be no history of acute spine pain, numbness, tingling, or muscle weakness. On physical examination, there should be no tenderness to firm palpation of the spine, and distal motor and sensory function should be fully intact.

The motor exam evaluates muscle function in the upper extremities by testing the strength of finger abduction (spreading fingers apart) or wrist extension against resistance. In the lower extremity, motor function is tested with plantar (towards the sole of the feet) and dorsi-flexion (towards the top of the foot) of the feet or big toes. Sensory function is assessed by the patient's ability to distinguish between sharp and dull touch on all four distal extremities.

A clear spine assessment means that there is no significant spine injury, and no need for spine stabilization. Any positive findings during the exam, such as tenderness or the inability to move the extremities equally, means that you should treat for spine injury. Later examination during evacuation or in the hospital may clear the spine, but for now you are obligated to stabilize the spine as best you can under the circumstances you're operating in.

It is important to note that many patients who have been involved in accidents on the highway, rocks, or ski slopes develop lots of minor aches and pains as swelling and inflammation increases over several hours. A stiff neck is one of these common late occurring symptoms. Because you were able to clear the spine initially and have not dropped your patient on her head since, this new onset of pain does not warrant stabilization.

TREATMENT FOR SPINE INJURY

When the spine cannot be cleared, note the reason on your problem list. Stating that the spine cannot be cleared due to neck tenderness or a neurologic deficit is useful in determining the sense of urgency and direction of evacuation. The ideal treatment for all spine injury is stabilization in normal anatomic alignment until the patient can be further evaluated on the trail or in the receiving medical facility. Stabilization can be accomplished with a variety of devices but requires some form of whole-body packaging. For backcountry rescue, this usually means an improvised or commercial litter.

While awaiting the proper equipment, a patient can be stabilized on a foam pad on the ground with packs or other gear positioned to restrict head motion. For evacuation times exceeding an hour, any device must be well padded with the patient in a position

of comfort with the knees bent. The patient must be monitored for symptoms of developing pressure sores. Hard backboards are a notorious problem in this regard.

The stiff extrication collars typically employed by EMS services are unsuitable for prolonged use. Acceptable cervical stabilization can be accomplished with clothing and other padding. The old ski patrol horse collar technique using a blanket, sleeping bag, or jacket, is effective, comfortable, and warm.

In packaging a patient for spine stabilization, the medical officer must be alert to anything that can cause ischemia or abrasion. The continuous jostling during evacuation can turn a small abrasion into a new addition to your problem list. Check your patient for earrings, jewelry, belts, clothing, and equipment. In the ideal package, the patient would be stripped to one layer of polypro to minimize the risk of developing problems.

Body position is important, too. Allow for knee flexion and for the arms to fold across the chest in the position of comfort. If the patient is alert, leave the arms free for self-protection, nose scratching, and food handling. Positioning your patient on his side may be more comfortable as well as allowing for drainage of oral secretions and vomit.

A full vacuum mattress inside a basket litter represents an ideal spine stabilization package for backcountry rescue. Depending on the mattress, additional cervical stabilization may not be necessary. It provides rigid stability and thermal insulation while conforming to the patient's contours.

Other devices such as a SKED, confined space litter, or improvised litter offer less flexibility for patient positioning. On a long evacuation, you may need periodic rest stops during which the patient is allowed to shift position and flex extremities. You should plan to do this for your patient if she is unable to do it for herself.

Whatever material or device you use, it should maintain normal spinal alignment in a comfortable and well-protected patient. A long evacuation will test the structural integrity of any package that you construct. Even the best of them will need adjustment

WARM 2008

Spine Injury Treatment
Spine cannot be cleared

Field Treatment:

• Restore spine alignment

• Package for protection and stability

• Treat pain, monitor for change

• Evacuate

and improvement along the trail.

WILDERNESS CONSIDERATIONS: SPINE STABILIZATION

There are situations in wilderness and technical rescue where the risk of spine stabilization exceeds the presumed benefit. Examples include patients or rescuers threatened by a wild-land fire, avalanche, or immersion hypothermia. In unstable scenes, the remote possibility of exacerbating a spine injury may not justify the additional risk associated with spine stabilization.

When you have no choice but to move immediately, you can take some comfort in the knowledge that unstable spine injury is very rare and the probability of further injury is remote. Remember, we are modifying the plan, not the diagnosis. Try to maintain alignment during rapid extrication if possible, and complete your stabilization as soon as the risk is minimized.

Another challenge to spine stabilization is an unsecured airway in a vomiting patient. In a rescue scenario, it can be extremely difficult to prevent aspiration of vomit, oral secretions, or blood into the lungs of an immobilized patient. It is sobering to realize that aspiration of vomit carries a mortality rate of 20 to 60%, depending on which studies are cited. It may be necessary to defer complete spine stabilization until you can reduce this high level of risk. In many cases, stabilization is best accomplished with the patient positioned on his side or in the recovery position.

The decision to defer stabilization to reduce some other risk may not be an easy one to make. The thought of a rescuer being responsible for permanent neurological deficit is appropriately frightening. However, the risk is minimal compared to the often substantial dangers of wilderness rescue and the morbidity and mortality associated with aspiration and other problems.

If you are forced to defer stabilization, the reasons should appear in your problem list. You might note that problem number one is a spine that cannot be cleared. Problem number two might be the fact that the temperature is 20 below zero with 30 knots of wind and you and your patient are at risk of freezing to death if you stay where you are.

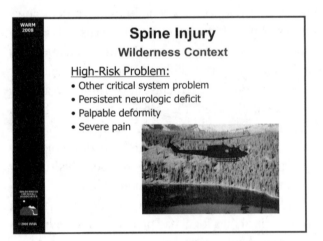

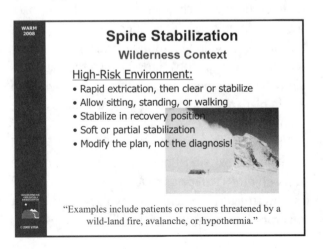

CASE STUDIES: CENTRAL NERVOUS SYSTEM

CASE #1

Scene: A 46-foot fishing vessel 50 nautical miles due east of Portland Head Light at 04:30. The weather was clear with winds of 15 knots, seas of 1 meter, and an air temperature of -3° C with light freezing spray.

S: A 40-y.o. fisherman was struck on the head while trying to secure a trawl door. This patient was found face down on deck within seconds of being seen upright at the rail. The unsecured gear was clear of the scene, and the patient's position was momentarily stable.

O: He was breathing and U on the AVPU scale for about 2 minutes before beginning to respond to questions. Once he was secure below decks, further exam showed swelling and discoloration on the back of his head, but no other injury. He complains of increasing headache and began to vomit after 30 minutes. Vital signs at 05:00:
P: 60, R: 22, BP: 140/72, S: cool, pale, T: 37.0 C Rectally, C: A on AVPU,
no memory for event, confused.

A: 1. Traumatic Brain Injury with increased ICP
         A': Severe increased ICP
      2. Vomiting
         A' dehydration
         A' airway obstruction
      3. Cold and Wet
         A' hypothermia
      4. Spine cannot be cleared because the patient is unreliable.

P: 1. Evacuation to neurosurgical care
      2. Recovery position, monitor airway
      3. Dry clothes, insulation, external heat source
      4. Maintain spine alignment as well as possible under the circumstances

Discussion: This is a nice, neat case for evacuation. The patient's signs and symptoms clearly indicate a high-risk problem, and the patient's mental status changes can be attributed to TBI with increased ICP. The patient was carefully monitored for any threat to the airway. The possibility of a helicopter evacuation was discussed with the Coast Guard, but the risk of dunking the patient in freezing water was considered to be too high. He arrived in port without incident.

Had this evacuation been prolonged, the crew would be concerned about maintaining hydration and calories for heat production. Advanced life support with IV therapy would become a priority, along with quick access to neurosurgical care. A helicopter pick-off might then be worth the risk.

CASE #2

Scene: 38-foot sailing vessel, 100 nautical miles south of Halifax, 13:00 hrs. Winds east at 20 knots, air temperature 15° C, water temperature 5° C, seas two meters from east, visibility unlimited.

S: During an uncontrolled jibe, the preventer fails allowing the boom to strike a crewmember on deck. The helmsman reports that patient was hit on the back of the head and knocked to the deck, but did not appear unconscious. The patient now complains of a headache and slight nausea. She has full memory for event. Denies allergies, is taking no medications, and has had no previous TBI. Her last meal was two hours ago.

O: Awake, cooperative, but uncomfortable. The examination finds moderate occipital scalp swelling with a four cm laceration. There is no palpable skull deformity. Bleeding is controlled by direct pressure. There is no neck or back tenderness, and no impairment of distal nerve function. The rest of the physical exam is unremarkable.
    P: 80, R: 16, BP: 118 by palpation, T: feels normal, Skin: wdp, C: Awake, alert, and oriented.

A: 1. Scalp laceration
            A': bleeding and infection
        2. Blow to the head
            A' Post concussive syndrome

P: 1. Clean and dress wound, monitor for infection, arrange medical visit at next port of call.
        2. Pain medication as needed. Monitor for food and fluid intake to prevent dehydration.

Discussion: There is no need for evacuation here. There is no traumatic brain injury and no risk of increased ICP. At home, of course, this patient would be seen in the emergency department, and her wound would be sutured. She may even have skull x-rays or a CT scan, depending on the level of concern for fracture. One hundred miles offshore, however, the risk of evacuation is not justified by the benefit of hospital treatment.

CASE #3

Scene: A hunting camp in the West Elk Wilderness, elevation 3200 meters. It is early November at 11:00 hrs. The weather is overcast with a 20 knot southwest wind and visibility of 100 meters in moderate snow. The air temperature is -5° C. Search and Rescue has taken four hours to reach the scene.

S: A 54--year-old hunter did not respond to breakfast call and is lying on his cot and refusing to get up. The guide reports that the patient drank a lot of whisky last night. His last known food and fluid intake was at 19:00 yesterday consisting of beans and sausage. His medical history unknown, but one of the other hunters reports seeing the patient taking some kind of pills, maybe vitamins.

O: The patient is found in a cold tent, half inside a sleeping bag wearing only long underwear. He is V on the AVPU scale, and verbal response consists only of garbled speech. He is shivering weakly. A bruise is noted below his right eye. No other obvious injury is found on exam, but a chest scar suggestive of open-heart surgery was seen. An inspection of his luggage and clothing finds a bottle of sub-lingual nitroglycerine tablets.

   VS: P: 100, R: 20, T: 33° C under the arm, Skin: pale, lips blue, C: V, disoriented BP: 102/62.

A: 1. Mild hypothermia
          A': severe hypothermia
      2. Compensated volume shock due to dehydration
          A': circulatory failure
      3. Low blood sugar
      4. Drug overdose (alcohol or other)
      5. Traumatic Brain Injury
          A': elevated ICP
      6. Hypoxia from cardiogenic shock due to myocardial ischemia
          A' circulatory failure

P: 1. Wrap to reduce heat loss
      2. IV hydration with warmed Normal Saline
      3. IV D50 or oral glucose
      4. Monitor for vomiting
      5. Consider evacuation options

Discussion: This is the value of the STOPEATS mnemonic. Although we can identify a most likely cause of his change in brain function, we must consider the full differential diagnosis. We then treat for what we can, and consider evacuation for what we cannot. In this case, the patient recovered with rewarming and hydration. He was able to assure rescuers that the bruise under the eye was from an earlier and unrelated event, and that he had, in fact, been taking vitamins and has not needed his nitroglycerine for several years. The patient refused evacuation, but agreed to sit out the hunt for a day to recover.

NOTES:

Basic and Advanced Life Support

8

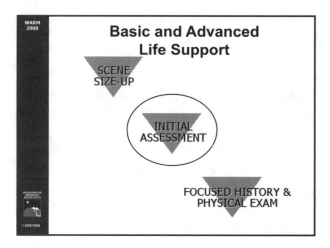

Basic Life Support (BLS) is the immediate treatment of life-threatening critical system problems discovered during the initial assessment. In terms of saving lives, the circulatory and respiratory components are equally important. Although BLS is outlined in a specific sequence, field treatment requires flexibility. It is often necessary to change the order in which things are done or to manage several components at the same time. The primary goal is to support oxygenation and perfusion of the brain and other vital organs.

Where available, Advance Life Support (ALS) is also part of the immediate response to life-threatening critical system problems. ALS techniques are more invasive, using a broad range of medications, advanced airways, and some surgical techniques. However, the goals of BLS and ALS are the same: to preserve oxygenation and perfusion.

Some techniques that were previously reserved for advanced level practitioners have been added to the basic scope of practice. The time-critical treatments for anaphylaxis and asthma offered in the protocols for wilderness medicine are examples. The use of automatic external defibrillators in the urban context is another.

At any level of medical expertise, it is important to understand what the next step along the chain of medical care should be. This allows for better referral and evacuation decisions. The BLS provider should know when ALS care may be beneficial, and conversely, when it isn't. If you know what type of care the patient needs, you may refine evacuation decisions and routes based on services available at one hospital or another.

BLS/ALS – RESPIRATORY SYSTEM

Your immediate response to respiratory failure or arrest is to ensure a patent airway, begin positive pressure ventilation, and apply any specific treatment that may necessary. This will be easier if you are able to identify what part of the respiratory system seems to be affected. As long as the heart is still beating,

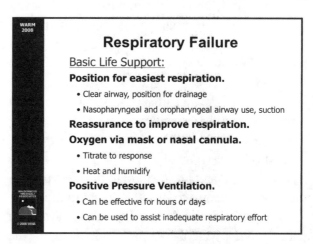

PPV can help to maintain oxygenation for many hours as assessment continues and the patient is evacuated to definitive care. The assessment criteria are pretty simple; if you don't think your patient is breathing well enough, begin PPV.

You can apply PPV directly with mouth to mouth, as is still taught in many CPR courses, but a mask or other barrier device should be used whenever possible. This is part of universal precautions and serves to protect both you and your patient. A pocket mask with filter and one-way valve is an essential part of any emergency medical kit.

The rate of ventilation should be about twelve breaths per minute. If you are unable to keep count, just start the next breath as soon as the patient has finished exhaling. Blow in enough air to cause the chest to rise slightly. Each breath is done slowly over two to three seconds. Faster flow rates tend to blow air into the stomach, causing distension and vomiting.

Patients who are breathing on their own, but not deeply or frequently enough, can still be assisted with PPV. This is especially useful in treating inadequate respiration due to chest wall injury or decreased nervous system drive. Timing your PPV to the patient's efforts is not critical; a patient in trouble will quickly adjust.

If you are unable to get air into the lungs, the problem may be upper airway obstruction. You may have already found clues to the mechanism in your scene size-up, such as an unfinished meal. Other causes of obstruction include swelling, spasm, position, and deformity from trauma.

Airway obstruction may be complete or partial. Complete obstructions will be rapidly fatal if not corrected. Partial obstructions tend to become worse over time, especially if aggravated by treatment. Do not attempt to clear a partial obstruction in the field unless it is causing respiratory failure.

Clearing an airway obstruction is a progression of actions from simple to desperate. Try to open the airway using a jaw thrust, chin lift, or direct pull on the tongue. Attempt to maintain in-line position on the head and neck to protect the spinal cord in trauma patients. If this type of positioning does not clear the airway, look inside the mouth. You may see a foreign body that can be pulled out with your fingers or a clamp.

If there's nothing to see, try using residual air to help clear obstructions. This is known as the Heimlich maneuver, chest compression, or abdominal thrust and can be done with the patient supine or sitting. It really doesn't matter whether you are squeezing the abdomen or the chest, the effect is the same. The sudden thrust can force the air left in the patient's lungs out under pressure, blowing any obstruction out with it. If that does not work, try a firm back blow between the shoulder blades. This also applies intrathoracic pressure and can help dislodge an obstruction.

If the obstruction is caused by swelling of the airway, back blows and abdominal thrusts will not help. The only BLS treatment is to continue PPV in an attempt to force air past the obstruction while repositioning the neck for the best air flow. These patients will need advanced life support with medication or a surgical airway.

If the cause of the airway swelling is anaphylaxis, an injection of epinephrine can be lifesaving. This is part of the Wilderness Protocol for Anaphylaxis, an ALS technique taught to basic practitioners because these patients may not survive long enough to access ALS level care. Life-threatening lower airway constriction due to asthma can be treated with epinephrine and steroids. This procedure is part of the Wilderness Protocol for Asthma, also taught to basic level practitioners for the same reason.

BLS/ALS: CIRCULATORY SYSTEM CARDIAC ARREST

Chest compressions are used to support perfusion when the heart has stopped. Unlike PPV, chest compressions are effective only for a very limited time. If functional cardiac activity is not restored within a few minutes, the patient will not survive.

Cardiac arrest means the loss of effective heart contractions indicated by the absence of a pulse. Cardiac arrest results in immediate respiratory arrest and complete loss of consciousness. A patient who is at all responsive, breathing, or moving spontaneously is not in cardiac arrest.

The pulse can be very difficult to find under adverse field conditions where you may be working with cold hands in dangerous places. The pulse can

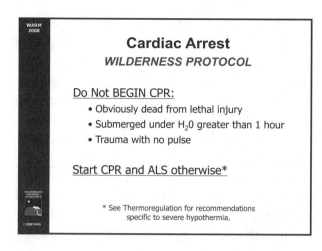

be weak or absent in the extremities of a person in shock, and very slow in profound hypothermia. It is extremely important to take the time to find a pulse. The carotid and temporal pulses are the easiest to get to, and always present if the heart is beating. The carotid is located on either side of the Adam's apple (larynx) in the neck. The temporal pulse is on the side of the head just in front of the ear.

Cardiac arrest is treated temporarily with cardiopulmonary resuscitation (CPR), which is a combination of chest compressions and PPV that allows some oxygenation and perfusion of the brain and vital organs. The technique has been learned by millions of people and has saved lives in settings where early defibrillation and ALS is available within a few minutes.

For CPR to be effective, the patient's critical systems must still be largely intact. CPR will not support perfusion in cases where the cardiac arrest was caused by massive trauma or shock. CPR will not work if the arrest was caused by brain or spinal cord injury.

The survivors of cardiac arrest are typically patients who have experienced ventricular fibrillation or other cardiac arrhythmia due to a heart attack. The lungs and brain are still intact and capable of resuming function if perfusion is restored. The application of electrical defibrillation within a few minutes of the arrest is occasionally successful in reestablishing normal cardiac rhythm.

In the United States and other developed nations, instruction in CPR is widespread, and automatic external defibrillators (AEDs) are now installed in airports and bus stations, and are being carried in police vehicles. The idea is to initiate CPR and defibrillation within the first few minutes while the heart has some chance of responding. Any reasonable chance of survival further depends on immediate access to ALS and a hospital. This system does save lives in urban areas. The best of such integrated medical systems have achieved cardiac arrest survival-to-discharge rates of around 20%.

Unfortunately, CPR has very limited application without access to a defibrillator, ALS, and hospital care. CPR by itself is unlikely to restore normal cardiac rhythm, and defibrillation alone will not fix the cause of the arrest. The chance of a successful resuscitation without definitive medical care is extremely low. To date, there are no documented saves using an AED in the backcountry or offshore setting.

Most of the successes attributed to CPR probably occur in cases where the heart was not actually in arrest. It is also possible that a cardiac arrest caused by respiratory failure, due to events like a near-drowning or lightning strike, could be reversed by prompt oxygenation of the lungs and chest compressions. How often this might occur is left to speculation. There are simply not enough monitored cases to know. We do know, however, that no one survives more than 30 minutes of CPR.

The Wilderness Protocol for Cardiac Arrest reflects our current level of experience and understanding. The chance of success does not justify any significant level of risk to survivors or rescuers. A backcountry evacuation with CPR in progress would be highly unusual.

Resuscitation should not be initiated when the cause of the arrest is trauma or severe blood loss, or the patient has been under water for more than an hour. Even when ALS techniques are used, resuscitation may be discontinued after 30 minutes of sustained cardiac arrest. Resuscitation can be discontinued at any time a cardiac monitor shows asystole, or an AED refuses to shock a pulseless patient.

SEVERE BLEEDING

Controlling blood loss is the other essential element of circulatory support in the BLS process. Bleeding from an artery is the most immediately life threatening and can usually be controlled by well-aimed direct pressure. The site must be exposed and the bleeding source identified. Direct pressure will be

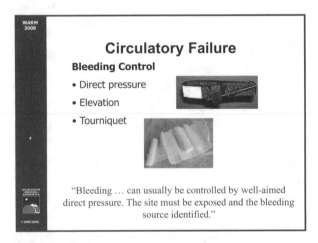

Circulatory Failure

Bleeding Control

• Direct pressure

• Elevation

• Tourniquet

"Bleeding … can usually be controlled by well-aimed direct pressure. The site must be exposed and the bleeding source identified."

effective most of the time if applied firmly enough, in the right place, and for long enough for the blood to clot.

A tourniquet may be used on an extremity to temporarily control severe bleeding while you deal with other critical system problems. It can also be used to stop bleeding long enough for you to expose and identify the source to better aim your direct pressure. A tourniquet can safely be left in place for up to an hour if necessary.

Pressure points, sometimes mentioned in first aid texts, are generally not effective for life-threatening

bleeding. Recently developed clot-enhancing powders that slow blood flow to allow for clot formation remain unproven in actual field use, and anecdotal experience is mixed. With abdominal gunshot wounds, clot enhancers may offer the only alternative treatment to try when direct pressure is ineffective.

No technique will work if you don't find the bleeding. Even profuse external bleeding can be hidden by snow and bulky clothing. This can be a real problem when the clothing is waterproof and the weather is too extreme to permit undressing the patient. A thorough exploration with a gloved hand is a mandatory part of the initial assessment of a trauma patient.

Internal bleeding is difficult to control without surgery. Some techniques, like binding a pelvic fracture, may reduce the space available for blood to accumulate. This tamponade effect may also stop internal blood loss in other confined spaces such as around the kidneys or inside the capsule of the spleen or liver. This fortuitous condition may allow time to evacuate the patient to surgery before shock progresses.

There are no ALS field techniques to control severe internal bleeding. In the presence of progressive shock, ALS providers may use IV fluids to maintain minimal effective perfusion pressure during evacuation (permissive hypotension). This must be done cautiously because increased pressure can disrupt clot formation, replacing the patient's blood with IV solution.

In treating shock from severe bleeding, access to IV therapy in the field is less important than access to replacement red blood cells and surgery. The practitioner should keep this in mind when making evacuation decisions. If the bleeding site is accessible and controlled, IV therapy may help to help maintain perfusion pressure and is less likely to be harmful.

BLS/ALS: THE NERVOUS SYSTEM

Abnormal brain function indicated by reduced level of consciousness or mental status changes can be caused by direct trauma to the nervous system or loss of brain oxygenation due to circulatory or respiratory system problems. There is no real way to treat this other than to treat the cause. BLS is aimed at protecting the airway from fluids and vomit, and the spine from further injury while assessment and treatment continues.

In trauma patients, the spine is stabilized as part of BLS. This takes the form of restoring and maintaining normal spinal alignment while treatment of any life-threatening condition continues. However, spine management should not take precedence over airway control, adequate ventilation, or circulatory support.

If you have to make a choice between a perfectly stable spine and an open airway, treat the airway. The benefits of breathing certainly outweigh the risks of spine injury.

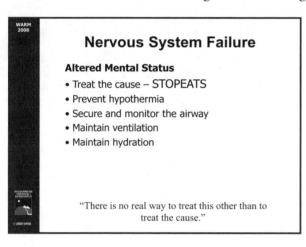

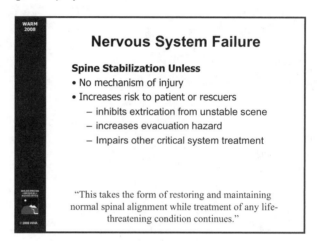

NOTES:

NOTES:

Allergy and Anaphylaxis

The severe systemic allergic reaction known as anaphylaxis causes major critical system problems that require immediate treatment in the field. The medications used are an important part of your BLS/ALS tool kit. The procedure should be memorized and rehearsed. This is a problem that will not wait for you to look it up in a book or for an ambulance or helicopter to arrive.

Allergy is an abnormal form of immune response resulting in the release of the chemical histamine into blood and body tissues. Histamine is a potent vasodilator and bronchoconstrictor. These effects can nearly instantaneous, or delayed by several hours.

When the response remains localized to the area of antigen contact, it is called a local reaction. The patient experiences localized vasodilation. This allows fluid to leak from capillaries into the extracellular space (fluid shift) causing swelling and itching. Hay fever is an example of a local reaction affecting the mucous membranes of the nose and eyes. The effects of histamine explain the familiar symptoms: swollen mucous membranes, itchy eyes, and a runny nose.

Anaphylaxis, by contrast, is a system-wide allergic reaction causing large amounts of histamine to be

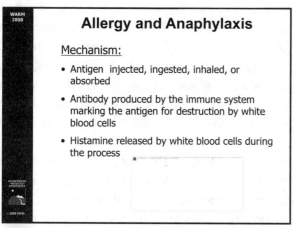

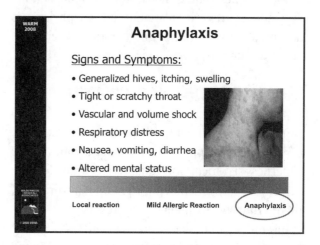

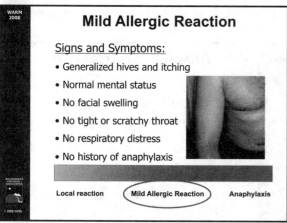

released into the general circulation. Hives, swelling, and itching develop throughout the body. The patient may give a history of a specific allergy, or the history may be completely unrevealing. A significant percentage of patients presenting with anaphylaxis will have no known history of allergy.

In its mild form, histamine response is characterized by generalized itching and hives with no swelling, no respiratory distress, and no signs of vascular shock. This mild allergic reaction often resolves on its own or responds well to treatment with oral antihistamines like diphenhydramine. Often, the patient will give a history of similar symptoms and

be mild or severe, local or systemic. Onset can be

successful treatment with oral medications. This is reassuring for field treatment, but still requires careful monitoring because any reaction can be more severe than expected.

Severe anaphylaxis, also called anaphylactic shock, is a major critical system problem. Widespread vasodilation and fluid shift can cause vascular and volume shock, upper airway swelling, and vomiting and diarrhea. Lower airway constriction results in wheezing and respiratory distress. The patient can die within a matter of minutes.

Initially, the patient may complain of itchy skin and hives with a scratchy or constricted feeling in the throat. Patients often report feeling a sense of impending doom. As the reaction becomes more severe, wheezing, stridor, facial swelling, nausea, vomiting, or diarrhea may develop. There will be weakness and mental status changes with the onset of vascular and volume shock. In the remote setting, early and aggressive treatment for anaphylaxis is warranted. This is especially urgent for a patient with a known history of severe anaphylaxis.

TREATMENT OF ANAPHYLAXIS

Specific ALS treatment with medication is required. BLS and PROP is appropriate, but not definitive. The Wilderness Protocol for Anaphylaxis calls for the use of the drugs epinephrine, diphenhydramine, and prednisone to immediately reverse the effects of histamine and block any reoccurrence of the problem. The recognition of severe anaphylaxis and the use of these medications is an important skill for the wilderness medical practitioner.

Epinephrine is a powerful vasoconstrictor and bronchodilator, temporarily opposing the effects of histamine. It is injected into the muscle of the shoulder or lateral aspect of the thigh at dose of 0.3–0.5 mg. The patient's symptoms usually improve within 90 seconds. Repeat doses may be necessary if symptoms do not improve or a rebound (biphasic) reaction occurs.

The epinephrine injection is followed immediately by an oral dose of 25-50 mg of diphenhydramine. This is an antihistamine that directly blocks the attachment of the histamine molecule to receptor sites on body tissues. Once it takes effect in 15–20 minutes, repeat doses of epinephrine should no longer be necessary. Other antihistamines can also be effective as an alternative to diphenhydramine.

Epinephrine is supplied as a liquid specifically for the treatment of anaphylaxis in the form of a pre-loaded EpiPen® or Twinject™ Autoinjector that automatically injects the right dose when pressed firmly against the skin. In the United States, these devices are available only by prescription. Patients known to have severe allergies often carry one. In the backcountry setting, it is advisable to carry at least three doses of epinephrine to cover biphasic reactions while the antihistamine is taking effect. Practitioners trained and comfortable with syringes and ampoules may choose to carry epinephrine in that more economical and compact form. Epinephrine should be protected from light, freezing, and excessive heat.

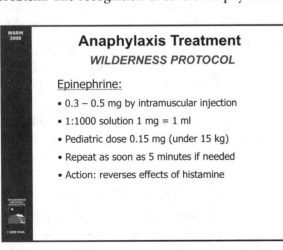

Anaphylaxis Treatment
WILDERNESS PROTOCOL

Epinephrine:

• 0.3 – 0.5 mg by intramuscular injection
• 1:1000 solution 1 mg = 1 ml
• Pediatric dose 0.15 mg (under 15 kg)
• Repeat as soon as 5 minutes if needed
• Action: reverses effects of histamine

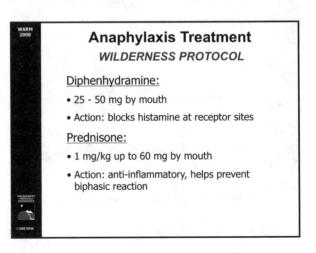

Anaphylaxis Treatment
WILDERNESS PROTOCOL

Diphenhydramine:

• 25 - 50 mg by mouth
• Action: blocks histamine at receptor sites

Prednisone:

• 1 mg/kg up to 60 mg by mouth
• Action: anti-inflammatory, helps prevent biphasic reaction

Diphenhydramine is supplied as a non-prescription medication in 25 mg tablets or capsules. A faster response may be obtained by using capsules and having the patient bite one open before swallowing. Warn the patient that the taste is very unpleasant.

Neither epinephrine nor diphenhydramine will remove the antigen or the histamine. It is possible to see a biphasic reaction with the reappearance of symptoms minutes to hours later. Continued use of the antihistamine for a day or so may be necessary.

For offshore situations or long evacuations, adding prednisone at a dose of 40–60 mg once a day may suppress the inflammatory response associated with the reaction. This will make a biphasic reaction less likely. Prednisone can be used at this dose for up to 5 days.

Because the effects of epinephrine are temporary, evacuation and medical follow-up should be planned.

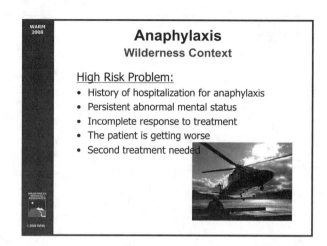

If the patient has recovered from the event, it need not be an emergency. Careful monitoring is crucial. A history of previous hospitalization for anaphylaxis or failure to improve to normal should motivate an emergency evacuation.

NOTES:

NOTES:

Asthma

Asthma is a chronic inflammatory disease that causes lower airway constriction. The mechanism involves both spasm of the smooth muscle walls and swelling of the mucous membrane lining of the bronchial tubes. Acute asthma attacks are sometimes triggered by infection, cold air, exercise, or other stressors. Sometimes asthma flares without apparent reason. Some patients need to use medications daily to keep their asthma under control.

An acute asthma attack can be mild or severe. It can be a major critical system problem when it causes respiratory distress. If bronchospasm is allowed

having it available at all. When early treatment is delayed or ineffective, the initial bronchospasm in the lower airways is made worse by secondary swelling. At this point, it will be difficult or impossible to deliver inhaled medication to the bronchioles where it can exert its effect.

Severe respiratory distress can rapidly progress to respiratory failure. At this stage, respiration will be labored with the patient only able to speak one or two words between breaths. Emergency treatment is required. This will not wait for evacuation or for ALS to be brought to the scene.

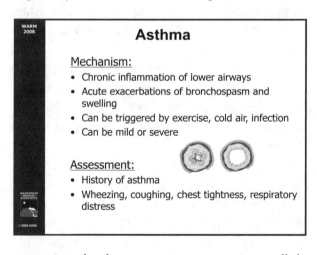

to persist, the lower airway constriction will be exacerbated by secondary swelling.

Early signs and symptoms include respiratory distress, chest tightness, wheezing, and a non-productive cough. Most people with asthma are aware of the condition and familiar with its presentation. Acute symptoms are usually relieved with self-administered medication like an inhaled beta-agonist (e.g., albuterol) that reverses the characteristic bronchospasm.

Occasionally, an asthma attack will not respond to inhaled medication. This is usually due to the patient's waiting too long to administer it or not

You should first assist your patient in the proper use of his metered dose inhaler (MDI). Be sure that you are using the fast acting bronchodilator. The patient may recognize this as his "rescue inhaler." The distinction is important because some patients also use an inhaled corticosteroid or other medication as an adjunct to therapy. These do not act fast enough to help in an acute attack.

Encourage the patient to inhale as deeply as possible while the inhaler is discharged into the mouth. The efficiency of the inhaler can be improved by the use of a spacer to contain the vapors while the patient inhales. This is simply a plastic tube with the

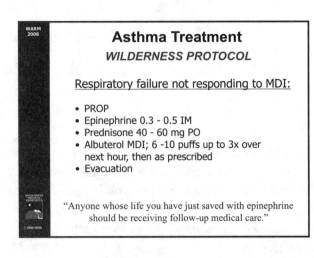

Asthma Treatment
WILDERNESS PROTOCOL

Respiratory failure not responding to MDI:

- PROP
- Epinephrine 0.3 - 0.5 IM
- Prednisone 40 - 60 mg PO
- Albuterol MDI; 6 -10 puffs up to 3x over next hour, then as prescribed
- Evacuation

"Anyone whose life you have just saved with epinephrine should be receiving follow-up medical care."

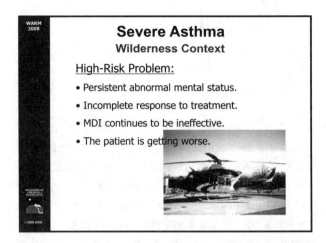

Severe Asthma
Wilderness Context

High-Risk Problem:

- Persistent abnormal mental status.
- Incomplete response to treatment.
- MDI continues to be ineffective.
- The patient is getting worse.

inhaler on one end and the patient on the other. You can improvise a spacer by using a plastic water bottle with the end cut off. Once the patient has inhaled the medication as deeply as possible, have him hold the medication in for a few seconds before exhaling.

It is safe to make several attempts to abort the asthma attack with an inhaler. However, do not delay moving to the next step if it is apparent that the patient cannot cooperate. If use of the inhaler fails to reduce symptoms within a few minutes, the patient will need an injection of epinephrine.

Before Beta-agonists like albuterol became available, epinephrine was a first-line treatment for an asthma attack. It is the same medication used for the emergency treatment of anaphylaxis. It is given in the same concentration and dose, and by the same intramuscular injection route.

The Wilderness Protocol for Severe Asthma calls for 0.3–0.5 mg injected into the muscle of the shoulder or lateral aspect of the thigh. The patient will usually feel better within a few minutes. One dose of epinephrine

may completely abort the asthma attack, but a second dose may be given within as little as five minutes if needed. Once symptoms improve, the patient should self-administer his own MDI. If evacuation is impossible or prolonged, add a dose of prednisone at 1mg/kg given by mouth (40–60 mg for an adult, 20 mg for a child). As with anaphylaxis, this will reduce lower airway inflammation and the chance of another attack.

Anyone whose life you have just saved with epinephrine should be receiving follow-up medical care. If the symptoms are under control, this need not be an emergency. A safe, monitored evacuation is appropriate.

This protocol is for use in severe respiratory distress caused by lower airway constriction in a known asthmatic. It is safe, effective, and carries little risk compared to the problems associated with prolonged respiratory distress. It is an important life-saving skill for both basic and advanced practitioners operating in remote areas.

Hypoglycemia

11

Diabetes has become a common chronic medical problem, and practitioners in any environment are likely to see a diabetic patient at some point. Fortunately, most diabetics are well-informed and do a good job of managing their disease. It is very likely that your diabetic client or traveling partner will know much more about it that you do. It is worth having a pre-trip discussion with the patient about anticipated problems and the appropriate treatment.

Diabetes is, in basic terms, the inability to produce the appropriate amount of insulin in response to rising blood sugar levels in the blood. Insulin is a hormone produced in the pancreas. One of its primary jobs is to help facilitate glucose uptake into body cells where it is processed and stored for use as fuel. When your patient eats, blood sugar rises as it does with everybody, but insulin levels do not. Insulin is usually injected or inhaled in a prescribed amount to match the caloric content of the meal.

Patients often adjust the amount of insulin and sugar intake in response to changing environmental conditions and activity. Most can monitor blood sugar any time with a portable glucometer. It is rare for a conscientious diabetic patient to get into trouble while living within a well-established routine.

Unfortunately, many backcountry and marine situations are far from well-established routine. Even a well-controlled diabetic can have trouble adjusting to a new environment. The problem is almost always low blood sugar, also known as *hypoglycemia*.

The symptoms of hypoglycemia can develop rapidly and usually start with mental status changes. Your patient may be normal one minute and become irritable, forgetful, or otherwise inappropriate the next. If not corrected, the patient can become combative, completely disoriented, or lose consciousness. Tachycardia and profound sweating are also commonly seen. Hypoglycemia is sometimes mistaken for intoxication or traumatic brain injury, delaying treatment until it is too late.

You are much less likely to see the opposite problem: hyperglycemia. The problem of too much sugar in the blood develops slowly over hours or days. Signs and symptoms include frequent urination, extreme thirst, weakness, and a fruity odor on the patient's breath. Most diabetics are aware that it is happening and will adjust their insulin dose accordingly, or seek medical care before serious problems develop.

TREATMENT OF HYPOGLYCEMIA

A diabetic with altered mental status is considered to be hypoglycemic until proven otherwise. The treatment is to administer easily absorbed sugar. For the patient who is still awake, the easiest route is orally in the form of a glucose gel kept in a first aid kit for that purpose. One dose is 15 grams of sugar. It is also fine to give granulated sugar, honey, candy, juice, or any other sweet food. Needless to say, sugar substitutes like saccharin will not work.

If the patient's level of consciousness has decreased to the point where airway protection is a concern, intravenous sugar is preferred. If IV therapy is not available, glucose, honey or granulated sugar can be rubbed on the mucous membranes inside the mouth where some will be directly absorbed into the blood. Sugar diluted in warm water or D50 can also be given rectally in the form of an enema.

Your unconscious patient may be carrying a glucagon injector. This is a kit containing a vial of powdered glucagon that is mixed with a solution, drawn up into a syringe, and injected into the upper arm, thigh, or buttocks. Glucagon is a hormone that increases blood sugar levels by releasing glycogen, a concentrated form of glucose, from the liver. Improvement should be seen within ten minutes. As the patient regains consciousness, sugar should be given orally.

If your client is carrying a glucagon kit, be sure that you examine it before you need it. Know where it is kept, and consider instructing someone else in the group in its use. Like epinephrine, a glucagon kit should not be allowed to freeze.

The administration of sugar, and glucagon if necessary, should result in rapid resolution of symptoms. If not, emergency evacuation should be initiated. Never give insulin to a diabetic with altered mental status, even if you have reason to believe that the problem is actually high blood sugar (hyperglycemia). The primary field treatment for that is aggressive hydration. You should also remind yourself of the STOPEATS mnemonic; low blood sugar may not be the only cause of the patient's condition.

Complete recovery from an episode of hypoglycemia ends the immediate emergency, but the practitioner must consider the patient's future safety. Can he reasonably expect to prevent another episode, and to effectively treat it if it does reoccur? As with other chronic conditions like asthma and angina, definitive treatment is a long way off if the emergency field treatment is not effective. It is possible that continued participation in a remote expedition may represent an unacceptable risk to the patient.

NOTES:

Section III
Trauma

General Principles of Trauma

12

ENERGY CAN NEITHER BE CREATED NOR DESTROYED

Kinetic energy is the energy of motion. When a moving object stops moving, its kinetic energy must be converted into another form or absorbed by the object and whatever stops it. The brakes on your truck, for example, convert the vehicle's kinetic energy into heat as you slow down.

Potential energy is possessed by an object waiting to fall. When the frost finally dislodges the rock above you, its potential energy is converted into kinetic energy. When the rock strikes your head, this energy has to go somewhere. Fortunately for you, the foam lining in your helmet absorbs the energy as it deforms, reducing the amount of energy transmitted to your head. Trauma happens when the human body absorbs enough kinetic energy to damage its structure, like the foam in your helmet.

KE=1/2 MV²

Kinetic energy is equal to mass times velocity squared, divided by two. This formula tells us that velocity contributes substantially more than mass to the kinetic energy possessed by a moving object. This explains how a very small, high-velocity bullet can do so much damage. It also tells us that a fast moving skier stopped by a large maple tree will dissipate a lot more energy than a skier moving only 5 mph slower. It explains why a fall from two meters in height may be no big deal, but four meters can be fatal.

DECELERATION

The rate of change in speed is called acceleration. Because injuries are usually caused by a sudden decrease in speed, or negative acceleration, we use the term deceleration. Deceleration requires the transformation or dissipation of energy over time.

When you step on the brakes, your truck does not decelerate instantly. There is time for the brakes to absorb and diffuse the truck's kinetic energy without damage to the vehicle or its occupants. If your truck were to decelerate instantly, against a bridge abutment, for example, massive deformation would result as the kinetic energy was absorbed instantly by the vehicle and the occupants. The difference between braking and crashing is the rate of deceleration.

Deceleration causes further injury due to inertia, the tendency of a moving body to keep moving until acted on by an outside force. If a skier's head is suddenly stopped by a maple tree, his brain would continue to move forward until it strikes the inside of the skull. This causes direct injury to the front of the brain from the impact and indirect injury to the back of the brain as suspended arteries and veins tear away from the brain tissue (also known as a contra-coup injury). The helmet might protect him from a skull fracture and scalp laceration, but it does little to prevent the brain from being injured by the sudden deceleration from high speed. The heart and great vessels can experience the same forces, resulting in a torn aorta.

Rapid deceleration concentrates energy and magnifies its effect. High kinetic energy with rapid deceleration causes the most damage. If your patient is a fast-moving skier stopped by a maple tree, you have a lot to worry about. This would be a good time to use the Big Net Principle in assessment.

By contrast, slow deceleration can dissipate a lot of energy without deforming structure. The high-speed skier who falls on a steep, open slope can dissipate his kinetic energy while sliding several hundred meters to a stop. He might even emerge uninjured. Ski patrollers call this a yard sale because ski equipment and clothing tend to dissipate as well. The skier's kinetic energy is actually converted into heat by the friction between his clothing and the snow. No deformation of his body was required to absorb the energy.

CAVITATION

High-velocity trauma can cause injuries remote from the point of impact due to an effect called cavitation. This is the sudden displacement of internal organs creating a shock wave that can distribute energy throughout the body. Low-density organs like the gut and lungs are elastic like foam rubber, and they can move and compress as they absorb the energy transmitted by cavitation. It is unusual to see rupture of hollow organs from blunt trauma.

High-density solid organs and bones are less elastic; they are more like watermelon and tend to split and fracture as energy is absorbed. This is how the spleen is ruptured by blunt trauma. There may be no visible external injury, but the solid organs inside can be shattered.

PAY ATTENTION TO THE HISTORY

Attention to the mechanism of injury and how kinetic energy was absorbed often gives you more information than the physical exam. For example, a patient who reports having the wind knocked out of him has just told you that his body has absorbed enough force to disrupt nerve function and possibly rupture internal organs. A sport climber whose fall was caught by a stretchy dynamic rope will have experienced substantially less deceleration than a rescue worker unfortunate enough to drop several meters on a static rope.

If your survey of the scene or history reveals a high velocity, rapid deceleration mechanism, you have good reason to suspect serious injury, perhaps remote from the site of impact. Trauma like this is more likely to involve shattered bone, ruptured organs, traumatic brain injury, and cardiac contusion. A thorough exam and careful monitoring is wise, regardless of the chief complaint and initial presentation.

Conversely, low velocity trauma tends not to cause injury elsewhere. It does not cause cavitation and deceleration is minimal. The initial damage is restricted to the point where the force is applied or where it is transferred by leverage or torque. In essence, what you see is what you get. In the patient with a complaint of knee pain following a slow twisting fall, you don't need to anticipate shock from solid organ rupture. In this case, the mechanism and history is reassuring.

Even when kinetic energy is high due to large mass, low velocity trauma is localized. The patient with a foot crushed by a ship rolling against the pier was exposed to massive kinetic energy by virtue of the size of the ship. But this is still a low velocity injury. No cavitation and no deceleration. The damage is all to the foot.

PROBLEMS ARE CUMULATIVE

An isolated injury to an otherwise healthy and safe individual is a rare delight in emergency medicine, especially in the backcountry. It is more common for trauma to be complicated by multi-system involvement, environmental extremes, and pre-existing injury or illness. A patient already in compensated volume shock from dehydration is not in a good position to survive fluid loss from a large burn. Mild hypothermia, by itself, can be cured in the field, but it vastly reduces the chance of survival for a patient in shock. Your problem list and plan must consider contributing factors beyond the acute trauma itself.

Extremes of age and chronic illness also elevate your level of concern. Elderly people are less able to compensate for volume loss due to less elasticity in the vascular system and reduced cardiac output. Small children lose heat much faster due to a larger surface area to weight ratio. Diabetics are going to have more difficulty maintaining oxygenation and perfusion of the extremities. A careful history can alert you to greater risk, or provide some degree of reassurance.

CRITICAL SYSTEMS COME FIRST

Major multi-system trauma can present a confusing picture. Assessment is complicated by acute stress reaction and the distractions caused by deformed fractures and pain. It is important to remember that musculoskeletal injuries and lacerations are never, by themselves, life-threatening problems. The severe bleeding associated with a femur or pelvis fracture is a circulatory system problem. Difficulty breathing in the presence of a rib fracture is a respiratory system problem. Altered mental status with a skull fracture represents a nervous system problem. Your initial assessment and basic life support should recognize and treat the critical system problems without being distracted by broken bones, pain, and superficial wounds. Trauma patients do not die of fractures, sprains, strains, and contusions. They die from shock, respiratory failure, and brain injury.

THE GOLDEN HOUR

The emergency medical services subscribe to the golden hour in trauma management as the ideal time within which the patient should access surgical care and stabilization. This is rarely possible in wilderness and offshore situations, but speed can still save lives. It is time to move fast if your scene survey or initial assessment reveals existing or anticipated critical system problems. Multiple-trauma patients need a hospital. In some situations, the focused exam will have to wait, perhaps even until the patient is out of the operating room.

HOLD THE FLUID

Experience in combat medicine from the beginning of the 20th century through the Vietnam War has demonstrated that aggressive fluid resuscitation of trauma patients in the field can be deadly more often than helpful. The intent in giving intravenous fluid to patients in shock is to maintain perfusion pressure and cellular oxygenation. Unfortunately, higher pressure within the circulatory system can also disrupt clot formation and exacerbate bleeding.

During recent conflicts in the Persian Gulf, American medics have been instructed to withhold IV fluid from casualties producing enough perfusion pressure to maintain A on the AVPU scale. If fluid was deemed necessary, it was provided with 25 ml boluses of hypertonic saline titrated to maintain peripheral pulses. Volume was not restored until operative control of bleeding was established in the hospital. Fatalities from major battlefield injuries fell to 12% from a century-long constant of 22%.

The implications for wilderness rescue are clear: for the trauma patient in shock from uncontrolled bleeding, IV fluid replacement is less of a priority than finding a surgeon and a hospital. If fluid replacement is performed, care should be exercised to avoid diluting blood and clotting factors with IV solutions. Maintaining body core temperature and rapid evacuation are much more likely to save a life than getting a blood pressure and starting an IV.

NOTES:

NOTES:

Musculoskeletal Injuries

If your survey of the scene and initial assessment reveals no existing or anticipated critical system problems, you have the luxury of time to perform a focused history and physical exam. You can develop a problem list and plan, and safely evacuate your patient to medical care hours or days later. Like most backcountry medical problems, musculoskeletal injuries are more often a logistical dilemma than any kind of emergency.

STRUCTURE AND FUNCTION

The structure of the musculoskeletal system is composed of bone, cartilage, tendon, ligament, muscle, and synovial fluid. Its function is support,

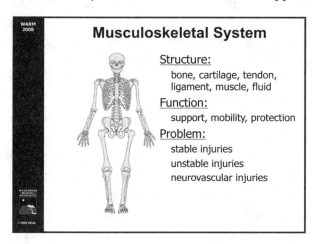

Musculoskeletal System

Structure:
bone, cartilage, tendon, ligament, muscle, fluid
Function:
support, mobility, protection
Problem:
stable injuries
unstable injuries
neurovascular injuries

protection, and mobility. The problems can be described generically as stable injury, unstable injury, and associated neurovascular injury.

Bone provides structural support and protection for soft tissue, and leverage for mobility. It is living tissue with a rich blood supply and an overlying membrane called the periosteum, which is abundantly supplied with sensory nerves. Like any other tissue, bones bleed and hurt when injured.

Bones meet at joints and are held together by

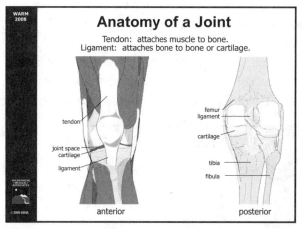

Anatomy of a Joint
Tendon: attaches muscle to bone.
Ligament: attaches bone to bone or cartilage.

tendon

joint space
cartilage

ligament

femur
ligament

cartilage

tibia

fibula

anterior   posterior

ligaments. Some joints are highly mobile, and some do not move much at all. Cartilage provides the smooth surface and padding where bones slide or pivot against each other. The synovial fluid contained inside the ligamentous joint capsule lubricates the surfaces.

Tendon is the cord-like connective tissue that joins muscle to bone, crossing joints in the cable and pulley system that effects movement. The muscle tissue itself is encased in connective tissue compartments called fascia. The steak you had for dinner offers a good cross section of this structure. The muscle is the soft red tissue and the *fascia* is the tough white grizzle that you don't eat.

Because muscle contraction is active and elongation is strictly passive, muscle groups must work in balanced opposition. One group is responsible for pulling a bone one way, and the opposite group is responsible for pulling the bone back. For example; the contraction of your biceps flexes your elbow and the contraction of your triceps extends it. Balanced opposition is an important concept to remember when splinting an injured joint or reducing a dislocation.

There are many types of bones and joints and many forms of injury. The mechanism can be direct or indirect force, overuse, infection, or even frostbite. Chronic conditions such as arthritis also affect structure and function. Knowing them in detail is interesting, but not required for effective field treatment.

Our primary concern will be whether an injured bone or joint can still safely perform its function or must be stabilized and protected. This is our generic assessment for the wilderness context: stable versus unstable.

When the structure and function of the system is compromised, surrounding soft tissue is also at risk. Of primary concern in extremity injuries are

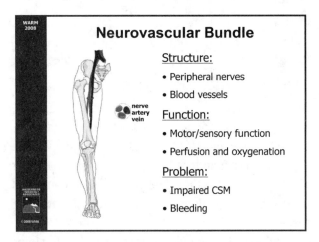

the arteries, veins, and peripheral nerves that run adjacent to bones and joints. They tend to be grouped in a ***neurovascular bundle***, much the way electrical wires and plumbing are fixed together as they run through a ship. These unprotected structures can be damaged during the initial injury or pinched by misalignment or swelling after the injury.

UNSTABLE INJURY

Fractures, sprains, and strains in extremities can be caused by a variety of mechanisms reflecting the different ways force can be applied to bones and joints. The injury may be caused by leverage, twisting, direct impact, or a piece of bone being pulled away at the site of attachment of a tendon or ligament.

High-velocity injuries, dissipating lots of kinetic energy in a short period of time, tend to cause ligament and tendon rupture and bone fractures. Low-velocity injuries are more prone to cause partial tears of ligament and tendon and are less likely to fracture bones. For field purposes, defining the mechanism of injury can be generalized to a yes-or-no question: Was there sufficient force to cause a fracture or rupture a ligament or tendon?

The signs and symptoms of an unstable

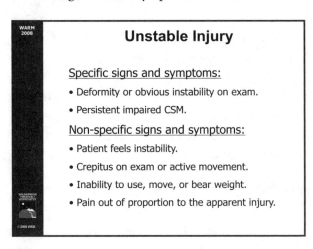

musculoskeletal injury are sometimes very obvious. Gross deformity, crepitis, and instability on exam make the assessment pretty clear. Also, the patient may report gross instability by telling you that his knee gives out every time he tries to walk. These criteria are very specific and indicate an injury that is definitely unstable.

Sometimes, you will have to rely on nonspecific signs and symptoms. Rapid swelling, for example, indicates significant bleeding at the injury site. The inability to use a joint or extremity after trauma indicates a more serious injury. Impairment of circulation, sensation and movement (abbreviated *CSM*) distal to the injury implies damage to the neurovascular bundle. The patient may report a snap or pop at the time of injury. Although these nonspecific criteria are less definitive, you might choose to treat the injury as unstable pending more information or response to treatment.

It is worth noting that the amount of pain is not a reliable sign. For example, a minor grade I ligament sprain will hurt much more than an unstable grade III ligament rupture. The primary pain receptors in ligaments are stretch receptors. Because the ruptured ligament is no longer being stretched, pain is minimal.

The primary complaint is often instability rather than discomfort.

It is important to stabilize any injury in which unstable fracture or ligament rupture may exist. Manipulation or use of extremities with fractured bones and loose or dislocated joints can cause further damage to surrounding soft tissue like the organs, muscles, and neurovascular bundle. This potential for damage is especially important to evaluate where the associated soft tissue is part of a critical system, such as the spinal cord running through damaged vertebrae or the femoral artery lying adjacent to a fractured femur.

Assessment for neurovascular bundle injury involves checking distal CSM. Problems with circulation are

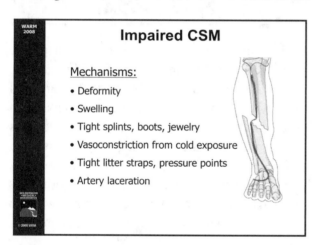

found by observing for signs of ischemia in the distal extremity, such as cool and pale skin, slow capillary refill, or a weak or absent pulse.

Problems with sensation are reported by the patient as numbness and tingling. Because nervous system tissue is exquisitely sensitive to oxygen deprivation, these are usually the first symptoms. The examiner can further evaluate the problem by checking the patient's ability to distinguish sharp from dull touch on the distal extremity. Often sharp and dull sensation is fully intact even with the complaint of numbness and tingling. The loss of motor control, such as wiggling fingers or toes, develops later in the course of ischemic injury. Ultimately, ischemic injuries can become very painful.

Extremity tissue can usually survive up to two hours

of ischemia with minimal damage. Beyond this, the risk of tissue death and permanent damage increases quickly with time. Ischemia also increases the risk of frostbite in freezing weather and makes infection more likely in open wounds. *If your treatment efforts do not succeed in restoring CSM, you have a limb-threatening emergency. Immediate evacuation is indicated if conditions permit.*

TREATMENT OF UNSTABLE INJURY

The process of stabilization has three distinct phases: traction into position, hands-on stable, and splint stable. Before you begin, check and document the status of the neurovascular bundle (check CSM). You will want to know that your treatment has improved the situation, or at least not made it worse. Most of the time, CSM will remain normal throughout the process.

Sometimes, an extremity feels numb or cold immediately following trauma, especially if a fracture or dislocation results in deformity, pain, and acute stress reaction. Your treatment should result in a significant improvement in CSM status as circulation is restored. Beware, however, that distal CSM may become impaired later as swelling develops under a splint or bandage. Detecting and correcting ischemia is an important function of continued care throughout your treatment and evacuation.

1. Traction into Position (TIP) – Injured bones and joints, and the soft tissues around them, are much more comfortable and much less likely to be damaged further if splinted in normal anatomic position. Although many injured extremities remain in good position or return there spontaneously, some will require manual realignment.

To restore anatomic position we first apply *traction*. This separates bone ends and reduces pain. Then, while traction is maintained, *position* is restored. Shaft fractures of long bones are returned to the "in-line" position where the effect of opposing muscles is most balanced and the neurovascular bundle is least likely to be compressed.

The amount of force necessary depends on the structure being realigned. Forearm and lower leg fractures usually require only gentle traction. Femur fracture, with the large surrounding muscle mass,

---

Unstable Injury
Long Bones

Treatment:

1. Traction Into Position
2. Hand Stable
3. Splint Stable
4. Check CSM before and after

TIP

"Your patient will be reassured to hear that traction into position is intended to be a slow and gentle process."

---

may require significant traction to restore length and alignment. Deformed wrist fractures may also require significant traction because of the way the bones ends tend to lock against each other.

Injured joints without dislocation usually do not need to be repositioned. If the patient is conscious and mobile, she will have already found the most comfortable position for the injured joint. If not, gentle TIP to a position in the mid range of the joint's normal motion will be most comfortable and put the least pressure on the neurovascular bundle. TIP may also be necessary to reposition a joint to allow for safe and stable splinting.

In joint dislocations, there is likely to be some loss of CSM distal to the injury. Under these conditions, TIP with movement toward the mid-range position is used until circulation is reestablished. In specific cases involving the shoulder, digits, and patella, TIP can be used to completely reduce dislocations with a significant improvement in comfort and circulation. The use of TIP on more complex dislocations, such as the elbow, wrist, or ankle is indicated only for restoration and preservation of circulation. Complete reduction of these dislocations may occur in the process, but is not an appropriate goal for field treatment unless the practitioner is very experienced with these types of injuries.

Spine injuries are also realigned by considering the stacked vertebrae of the spine to be a single long bone with a joint at the pelvis and the skull. However, traction should not be used. Spine alignment and

---

Unstable Injury
Joints

Treatment:

• Splint in position found
• TIP to reposition if...
  • CSM is impaired
  • Position impedes effective splinting or evacuation

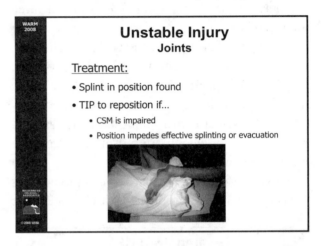

---

stabilization is discussed in more detail in Chapter 7.

Traction into position is a safe procedure if done properly. To be successful at reducing pain and restoring position, it is critical to have the cooperation and confidence of the injured person. Muscle groups in spasm or a patient fighting your efforts will vastly complicate the procedure. Your patient will be reassured to hear that traction into position is intended to be a slow and gentle process. It will also help to let her know that she is in control and that you will stop the process if she asks.

The therapeutic effect of a calm voice and reassuring manner is truly amazing. What this treats, of course, is the patient's acute stress reaction, as well as yours. Pain medication is valuable but can be dangerous to use in the backcountry setting at the dosage necessary to completely relax a scared and uncomfortable patient. Field treatment combining reassurance with the lowest effective dose of medication can offer less risk with equal benefit.

Open shaft fractures with bone ends protruding through the skin are still managed with TIP following thorough cleaning of the exposed bone ends and surrounding skin (see Chapter 14). To keep skin from becoming trapped under the bone as you realign the fracture, you may have to pull it free with forceps or gloved finger as the bone is manipulated back into the wound.

Occasionally it will be impossible to comfortably and safely restore position, even using TIP. You should discontinue TIP and stabilize the injury in the position found if TIP causes a significant increase in pain or resistance. These rare situations represent a limb-threatening emergency if deformity is significant or ischemia is detected.

2. Hand Stable – Once you have repositioned an extremity injury, stability must be maintained until the splint can take over. This may mean having someone hold gentle traction on the extremity while you prepare for splinting. If you are alone, you can use snow, rocks, or pieces of equipment to hold the limb in place.

3. Splint Stable – Whether a commercially manufactured product or something improvised from your equipment, a splint should be complete, comfortable, and compact.

Complete: Long bones should be splinted in the in-line position, and the splint should immobilize the joint above and below the injury. To effectively splint a lower leg fracture, the ankle and knee must be immobilized. Joint injuries are splinted in the mid-range position, including the bones above and below the injury. To splint the elbow, for example, the forearm and upper arm are included in the splint.

For splinting purposes, the stacked vertebrae of the spine may be viewed as a long bone with joints at the pelvis and base of the skull. Splinting a spine injury would require stabilizing the pelvis, shoulders, and head. Unstable pelvis injuries require stabilization of the spine and femur. Femur fractures require stabilization of the pelvis and knee. For these spine, pelvis, and femur injuries, the ideal treatment is whole-body stabilization in a litter or vacuum mattress.

Comfortable: Splints should be well padded, strong, and snug. There should be no movement of the injured bones or any pressure points or loose spots. It should allow you to monitor distal CSM, and be easily adjustable if ischemia or pain develops. A good splint decreases pain and preserves CSM. Attention to this principle is critical to prevent pressure sores and infection during long-term care and transport.

Compact: For wilderness use, a splint should be no larger or more complex than absolutely necessary. It should not inhibit the evacuation you have in mind. A simple sling and swathe, for example, splints everything from the clavicle to the elbow. This simple structure can be created with a safety pin and the patient's shirt. No additional material is necessary.

Once an injury is stabilized, the most important anticipated problem for long-term care becomes distal ischemia caused by compression of the neurovascular bundle as swelling develops inside splints or bandages. Treatment should include medication, rest, and elevation to reduce swelling and pressure. This is essentially the same as the generic treatment for stable injuries. As long as distal CSM remains normal or continues to improve, you can take your time planning a safe and comfortable evacuation.

SPECIAL CONSIDERATIONS FOR THE WILDERNESS CONTEXT

Femur Fracture – Shock and distal ischemia are anticipated problems due to the proximity of the neurovascular bundle to the femoral shaft. The usual treatment for a femoral shaft fracture in the EMS setting is the application of a traction splint and urgent evacuation to a hospital. This may be appropriate for short-term care, but the risks outweigh the benefit in long or difficult evacuations.

In many backcountry situations, it can be

impossible to distinguish a femoral shaft fracture from a femoral neck or pelvis fracture that might be further deformed by the application of traction. Even when properly applied, traction splints are notoriously difficult to monitor and package. When the proper amount of traction is applied to the femur, the pressure at the anchor points will inevitably cause skin and soft tissue ischemia. For these reasons, the use of a traction splint may not be appropriate or safe for backcountry rescue or long-term care. In this setting, femur fractures are best stabilized in a litter, vacuum mattress, or well-padded backboard.

Pelvic Fracture – Shock and distal ischemia are anticipated problems due to the proximity of the iliac arteries and veins. Pelvic binding with a padded strap or wide compression bandage may be useful to help stabilize a pelvic fracture and reduce the space available for internal blood loss. This can be accomplished by wrapping a tarp or backpack hip belt around the pelvis and tightening gently to restore anatomy. The patient is further stabilized by a litter, vacuum mattress, or well-padded backboard. Urgent evacuation is indicated.

Compartment Syndrome – Swelling due to bleeding or edema inside a muscle compartment can increase intra-compartment pressure to the point that perfusion is impaired. The mechanism is usually blunt trauma or collateral damage from a fracture. It is also possible to see compartment syndrome develop from repetitive motion injury. Ischemia develops, with

necrosis of muscle and nerve tissue as the anticipated problem. Symptoms include pain out of proportion to the apparent injury, distal numbness, and pain on passive stretching of the affected muscle group. Compartment syndrome can develop hours to days after the initial injury. Field treatment includes anti-inflammatory medication, rest, elevation, and cooling of the extremity. Urgent evacuation is indicated if immediate improvement is not noted.

Open Fracture – Fractures may be open (compound) or closed (simple). In an open fracture, the site is exposed to the outside environment through a wound in the skin. This opening can be produced from inside by sharp bone ends, or from outside by the same object that caused the fracture (like a bullet). Fortunately, open fractures are uncommon.

Distal ischemia and infection are anticipated problems. Aggressive debridement and cleaning are necessary before bone ends are pulled under the skin. Prophylactic antibiotics should be considered as part of the ideal field treatment. In cases such as crush injuries where bones remain exposed, moist dressings over the wound will help preserve tissue. Urgent evacuation is indicated.

Joint Infection – Also called septic arthritis. The symptoms of joint infection include swelling, redness, pain, and warmth. The patient may develop a fever. Joint infection usually develops shortly after a laceration or puncture wound that penetrates the joint space, but may develop after a minor abrasion or

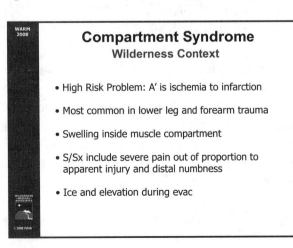

Compartment Syndrome
Wilderness Context

- High Risk Problem: A' is ischemia to infarction

- Most common in lower leg and forearm trauma

- Swelling inside muscle compartment

- S/Sx include severe pain out of proportion to apparent injury and distal numbness

- Ice and elevation during evac

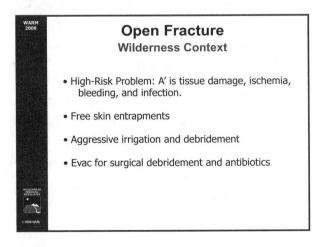

Open Fracture
Wilderness Context

- High-Risk Problem: A' is tissue damage, ischemia, bleeding, and infection.

- Free skin entrapments

- Aggressive irrigation and debridement

- Evac for surgical debridement and antibiotics

without any skin defect being visible. These infections have the potential to become systemic, and result in life-threatening vascular shock.

Impending Surgery – Serious fractures, infections, and compartment syndromes will be likely candidates for immediate surgery upon arrival at the hospital. For the anesthesiologist preparing the patient for surgery, vomiting is an anticipated problem associated with general anesthesia and intubation. For that reason, EMS personnel in the ambulance context do not give any fluids, food, or medications by mouth to such patients. This is referred to as keeping the patient *NPO*, an abbreviation for the Latin *nil per os*. Intravenous fluids and IV or IM medications are used instead.

During a long evacuation, priority must be given to maintaining hydration, perfusion, and body core temperature. Fluid replacement by intravenous line is ideal, but oral intake of fluids will be necessary if the IV route is not available or is impractical. Food is important in maintaining calories for heat production. You can help the anesthesiologist by giving your patient easily digested and absorbed simple sugars and carbohydrates, and avoiding protein and fat when possible. NPO is not an option in most prolonged evacuations.

STABLE INJURIES

Stable musculoskeletal injuries will have none of the specific signs and symptoms associated with instability. Often, the patient will have been able to move, use, or bear weight with the extremity within a short time after injury. There will be no history of instability. Any swelling will have developed slowly over several hours. You will find no deformity, crepitis on movement, or instability on exam.

Treatment is designed to reduce and control swelling and pain and includes using anti-inflammatory medication as well as rest, ice if available, compression, and elevation (RICE). Because a stable injury is safe to use within the limits of discomfort, the patient is allowed pain free activity.

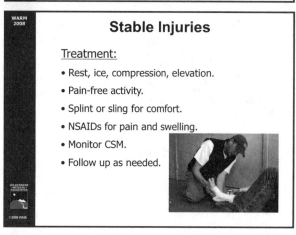

Stable Injuries

S/sx:
- No deformity, no instability on exam
- No sense of instability reported by patient
- Able to move and bear weight after accident
- Distal CSM intact
- Slow onset of swelling
- Pain proportional to apparent injury

Stable Injuries

Treatment:
- Rest, ice, compression, elevation.
- Pain-free activity.
- Splint or sling for comfort.
- NSAIDs for pain and swelling.
- Monitor CSM.
- Follow up as needed.

Elevation and rest are the most important elements of RICE, and most useful early on when the swelling is likely to be the worst. Ice is also very helpful. Even in the summer, you can achieve some cooling by evaporation by wrapping the injury in a water-soaked bandage.

Compression of an injured extremity with an elastic bandage is intended to limit the space available for swelling or to force accumulated fluid out of the extracellular space. Sometimes this is helpful, but it can also contribute to compartment syndrome and increase swelling of the distal extremity. Compression bandages may also be employed to provide some support to a sore joint. Frequent monitoring of the distal CSM is important when using a compression bandage.

Medication such as aspirin, ibuprofen, or acetaminophen can help reduce discomfort. A regular dose over several days will raise a good level of the drug in the body and may work better than just taking it occasionally in response to pain. Because aspirin and ibuprofen inhibit blood clotting and increase swelling from bleeding, acetaminophen may be preferred in the immediate post-injury period.

Pain free activity is allowed after the first 24 hours or when most of the pain and swelling has resolved. The patient may perform whatever activity is possible as long as pain is not increased. This may include skiing, or it may require very limited use around camp for several days.

Following these treatment guidelines, all stable injuries should show steady improvement. If not, your patient is being too active or your assessment may be wrong. It is possible to have a stable injury with a small fracture causing prolonged discomfort. Medical follow-up is indicated if rapid improvement is not noted or symptoms persist at the end of the trip.

OVERUSE SYNDROMES

Bursitis, tendonitis, and joint inflammation can be symptoms of overuse. These injuries develop over time without an obvious precipitating traumatic event other than repetitive motion. A long hike or bike ride can bring on pain and near-complete disability. You should be able to rule out unstable injury by history, but that may not make the patient any more functional.

You will note pain, swelling, and sometimes redness over an inflamed muscle, tendon, or joint structure. Moving it will hurt, and you may be able to feel crepitis as a damaged tendon slides roughly through an irritated tendon sheath. Resting it will feel better. These symptoms are typical of all kinds of repetitive motion injury. Bikers get it in the knee, hikers in the foot, and rowers in the wrists.

To effectively treat an overuse syndrome, you have to break the cycle of injury and inflammation. Treatment includes RICE and anti-inflammatory medication. If travel is required, functional splinting for support and mobility will be necessary. As pain subsides, remove the splint two or three times a day and do gentle exercises taking the part through its

normal range of motion as pain allows. Apply heat after the initial inflammation has settled down. Use warm soaks four times a day for 15 minutes at a time. This is good to do just before range of motion exercises.

In order to keep moving, change the way your patient performs the repetitive motion. This will put the stress on different muscle/tendon groups. For example, using a short loop of webbing as a handle on a kayak paddle can allow you to pull with your wrist held vertically instead of horizontally. This may not be ideal, but it may allow the group to continue travel.

Take the full therapeutic dose of anti-inflammatory medication. For ibuprofen, this is 3200 mg a day. You can minimize gastrointestinal and kidney problems by taking these drugs with lots of water and food. Your stomach may allow a couple of days of this, which can suppress the inflammation enough to prevent complete disability. Reduce the dose as soon as improvement is noted.

Using tape and padding, you can create a soft splint that will help reduce the stress on the irritated structure. Joint taping is another technique for providing support and limited mobility. Rest frequently, letting pain be the signal to stop. Continue only after it is under control.

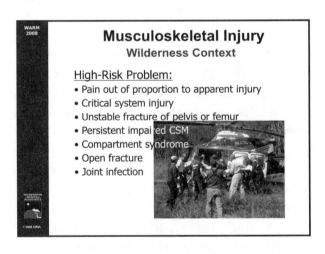

Musculoskeletal Injury
Wilderness Context

High-Risk Problem:
- Pain out of proportion to apparent injury
- Critical system injury
- Unstable fracture of pelvis or femur
- Persistent impaired CSM
- Compartment syndrome
- Open fracture
- Joint infection

CASE STUDIES: MUSCULOSKELETAL SYSTEM

CASE #1

S: A 43-year-old backcountry guide was skiing a late spring snow field when he caught an edge, causing a tumbling fall. He felt a pop and a brief burning pain in his left knee. On attempting to stand, the knee "gave out." He did not hit his head and has no neck pain. He had full memory for the event. He has an allergy to vicodin, takes ibuprofen for headaches, has never injured the knee before, and has no significant past medical history. His last meal was 40 minutes ago. The descent was at the end of the day, with only a half mile to go. He had attempted to ski further, but the left knee "gave out" when he tried to turn.

O: The guide was found sitting upright in stable position with the left knee flexed. He was fully alert, warm, and reasonably dry. He had no spine tenderness. The left knee was tender but not swollen, deformed, or discolored. He was able to flex and extend the knee fully with little discomfort. Distal CSM was intact. There was no other obvious injury. Vital Signs at 13:20 were normal.

A: 1. Unstable injury left knee
 A': Distal ischemia due to swelling

P: The knee was stabilized by an improvised litter fashioned from ensolite pads and nylon webbing. Despite his embarrassment, the man was carried the last half mile to the road. Distal CSM was monitored by asking him if he could feel and wiggle his toes inside his boots.

Discussion: Although the temptation to limp the last half mile was very strong, the patient agreed to the appropriate treatment. This injury fit the criteria for unstable injury because of the history of a "pop" during injury and the instability experienced afterwards. This story is typical of an anterior cruciate ligament rupture.

CASE #2

S: A 17-year-old girl caught her right index finger between loose rocks during the descent of a talus slope fifteen miles from the trail head. She was able to dislodge herself, but complained of immediate pain. Shortly afterward, she became dizzy and nauseous. The group leader climbed back up to examine the girl. Witnesses told him that she did not fall and was not struck by anything. She has no allergies, is not on medication, and has no significant past medical history. She had breakfast 1 hour ago. She had been walking without difficulty prior to the accident and was well rested and hydrated. The rock was stable but the weather was cool and windy.

O: The patient was found lying against a large rock. She was disoriented, pale, and sweaty. The right index finger was very tender with obvious deformity at the proximal interphalyngeal joint. The patient was unable to demonstrate any range of motion. There was no other injury. Her Vital Signs at 09:30 were—BP: unknown, P: 64, R: 24, Skin: pale, cool, moist, T: feels cool, C: V on AVPU with confusion and disorientation, improving.

A: 1. Dislocation right index finger
      A': Swelling and ischemia right index finger
  2. Acute Stress Reaction

P: The finger was immersed in a cold stream to relieve pain. The joint was reduced with minimal traction. She was encouraged to lie in a sleeping bag and calm down. Her vital signs rechecked at 10:00 were normal. The finger was splinted by taping it to the third finger with a gauze pad between the fingers.

    The girl was instructed to keep the finger elevated as much as possible and use cool soaks for swelling and pain relief during rest stops. She was cautioned to check circulation and sensation at the fingertip frequently. She would be referred to medical care when the group reached the road in three days.

Discussion: Although this patient was displaying very frightening signs and symptoms immediately after the injury, there was no mechanism to explain it, except ASR. The changes in mental status rapidly resolved with rest, reassurance, treatment, and pain relief, leaving only an unhappy girl with a sore finger.

Joint Dislocations

14

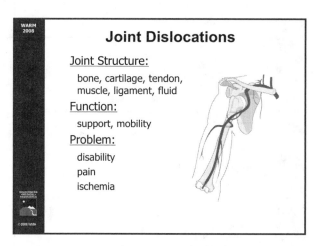

Joint Dislocations

Joint Structure:

bone, cartilage, tendon, muscle, ligament, fluid

Function:

support, mobility

Problem:

disability
pain
ischemia

A joint is a complex assembly of bones, ligaments, cartilage, tendon, muscle, and synovial fluid. These structures can be injured in a wide variety of combinations and levels of severity. A dislocation occurs when enough force is applied to the bone to tear the restraining ligaments and allow the joint to come apart. Using traction into position to restore a joint to normal anatomical position is called reduction.

There are three specific dislocations that are easy and safe to reduce in the field; the shoulder, patella, and digits. The Wilderness Protocol for Joint Reduction is for use in situations where the mechanism involves low-energy and indirect force. With proper technique, the medical officer can transform a gruesome and painful medical emergency into a minor logistical problem.

In cases where the deformity is the result of high kinetic energy, such as a long fall on a rock face or high-speed ski accident, a dislocation is more likely to be complicated by fractures and other injury. Reducing a dislocation under these circumstances involves more risk. Splinting in place and urgent evacuation is ideal.

SHOULDER DISLOCATIONS

The usual mechanism for simple dislocation of the shoulder is forced external rotation and abduction such as high-bracing with a kayak paddle or catching a fall on an outstretched arm while skiing. The velocity is usually low, and the mass is restricted to the weight of the patient. Fractures are uncommon, and generally do not interfere with treatment.

Shoulder dislocations can be extremely uncomfortable, and there is often some degree of CSM impairment. Acute stress reaction is common. The shoulder itself loses the contour of the deltoid muscle and becomes a step off deformity, with a hollow area where the shoulder is normally full and rounded. The patient will lose active range of motion, that is, be unwilling to move the shoulder joint without help.

Occasionally, a shoulder dislocation can be confused with a shoulder separation, which is a disruption of the joint between the distal end of the clavicle (collar bone) and the scapula (shoulder blade). The usual mechanism of injury is a direct blow to the top of the shoulder during a fall.

This joint lies directly above the shoulder joint and can have a similar step off appearance caused by the displaced and elevated distal end of the clavicle. However, the shoulder joint itself retains active range of motion and the rounded deltoid contour.

TREATMENT OF SHOULDER DISLOCATION

The damage to the joint and surrounding soft tissue due to ischemia will increase significantly after a couple of hours. A simple dislocation of the shoulder should be reduced in the field if the evacuation time to definitive care will be greater than two hours, or the evacuation will be difficult or dangerous to perform while the shoulder remains displaced. These criteria apply to most backcountry and marine situations.

There are a number of techniques that are effective in reducing dislocated shoulders. The best we've found for field use requires only a small patch of level ground and one rescuer. Because it is performed gently and slowly, it carries a low risk of causing further injury. The patient's cooperation and relaxation is essential.

To begin, the patient's arm is supported while he is being helped into a position lying on his back. Gentle traction on the upper arm will help relieve pain during movement. Lying the patient down may take some time. Once the patient is supine, the rescuer slowly abducts and externally rotates the arm into a position about 90° from the body, with the elbow bent. It is exactly the position the patient would have his arm if he were about to pitch a hardball. Once the arm is in position, make yourself comfortable and begin to apply steady traction.

Traction should be firm, but there should be no need for counter-traction unless you are working on ice or snow. The patient should be gently and repeatedly encouraged to relax his shoulder muscles. Usually, within a few minutes, the muscles will fatigue allowing the joint to slip back into place. If nothing has happened after about 15 minutes, try a move called throwing the baseball. This movement is exactly like it sounds.

Watch the patient's shoulder and pick a moment when you see the muscles really relax. Gently rotate the arm and hand forward as if the patient were throwing a ball. This is almost always successful in encouraging the shoulder to pop back into its socket.

Another safe technique for field use is scapular manipulation. Instead of rotating the humeral head into place in the socket, we slide the socket into place behind the humeral head. Traction and external rotation is applied to the humerus by an assistant, while the lower portion of the scapula is pulled medially by the rescuer. This drops the socket into place behind the humerus. As with the baseball

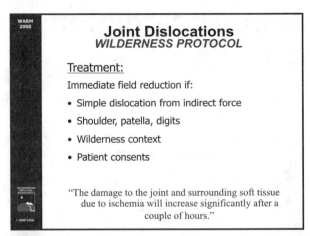

Joint Dislocations
WILDERNESS PROTOCOL

Treatment:

Immediate field reduction if:

- Simple dislocation from indirect force
- Shoulder, patella, digits
- Wilderness context
- Patient consents

"The damage to the joint and surrounding soft tissue due to ischemia will increase significantly after a couple of hours."

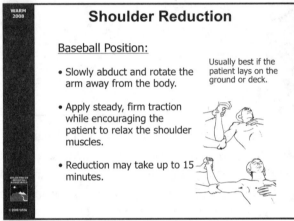

Shoulder Reduction

Baseball Position:

- Slowly abduct and rotate the arm away from the body.

Usually best if the patient lays on the ground or deck.

- Apply steady, firm traction while encouraging the patient to relax the shoulder muscles.
- Reduction may take up to 15 minutes.

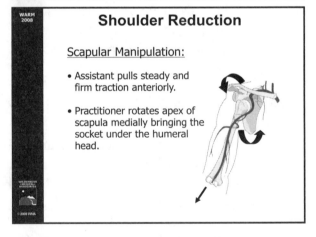

Shoulder Reduction

Scapular Manipulation:

- Assistant pulls steady and firm traction anteriorly.
- Practitioner rotates apex of scapula medially bringing the socket under the humeral head.

technique, slow and gentle manipulation with a relaxed patient will have the best chance for success.

You will recognize a successful reduction by the dramatic relief of pain and return of mobility. You can sometimes feel and see a sudden shift of the upper arm as it relocates in the socket. If CSM impairment was present before reduction, it will rapidly improve afterward. Remember to check and document CSM both before and after reduction. The most effective splint is a simple sling. The patient should plan for medical follow-up within a week, if possible. Pain free activity is safe as long as the patient avoids abduction and external rotation.

Some shoulders will remain quite painful immediately after reduction. This sometimes indicates that a small piece of bone is chipped off of the head of the humerus. This should not be a cause for urgent evacuation as long as distal CSM (particularly circulation and sensation) is intact. A sling with a swath to restrict movement may be more comfortable.

Dislocations that result from direct force are generally more complicated and usually not reduced in the field. Manipulation is directed only at restoring CSM, if necessary, and positioning the patient for safe evacuation. If the patient is to be walked out, a sling pinned to the patient's shirt or jacket is effective immobilization.

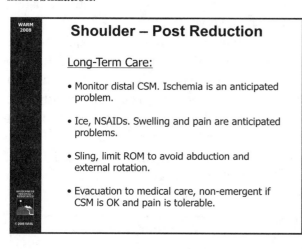

Shoulder – Post Reduction

Long-Term Care:

- Monitor distal CSM. Ischemia is an anticipated problem.

- Ice, NSAIDs. Swelling and pain are anticipated problems.

- Sling, limit ROM to avoid abduction and external rotation.

- Evacuation to medical care, non-emergent if CSM is OK and pain is tolerable.

PATELLA DISLOCATION

The patella (kneecap) is an isolated bone imbedded as a fulcrum in the quadriceps tendon. This large structure transmits the force of the contracting quadriceps muscle in the front of the thigh to the front of the lower leg to allow you to extend your knee. The tendon passes over a groove in the femur like a cable through a pulley. In patellar dislocation, the tendon and patella slips off the femoral groove making it impossible for the knee to function.

Like the shoulder, the patella can dislocate with a direct blow or indirect mechanism—typically a sudden extension of the knee while twisting or turning with the foot fixed in position by a crampon or ski. The patient often has a history of recurrent dislocation. An indirect dislocation always leaves the patella pinned against the outside of the knee by the pull of the quadriceps (a lateral dislocation). The appearance can be deceiving. Shifting the patella laterally will make the end of the femur on the inside of the knee stand out and look like the missing patella.

Like the shoulder, these dislocations also are extremely uncomfortable, and there is little or no active range of motion. Because the neurovascular bundle is not nearby, distal circulation and sensation is usually unaffected. Damage to other surrounding soft tissue will increase with time, as will the difficulty of reduction.

TREATMENT OF PATELLA DISLOCATION

Like the shoulder, a dislocated patella should be reduced if access to medical care will be delayed by more than two hours or the evacuation will be unreasonably difficult. Take the tension off the structure by sitting the patient up to flex the hip. Then slowly straighten the knee. If the patella does not reduce on its own, push it gently into place with your thumbs. Like the shoulder, relief of pain and return of mobility will indicate success. Also like the shoulder, these injuries are likely to result in swelling and significant pain later.

Ideally, a reduced patella dislocation should be splinted as an unstable injury and carried out. In less than ideal situations, the knee could be braced and the patient walked out if pain permits. Taping the patella to prevent lateral displacement is often effective. It is important to avoid repeating the mechanism of injury. As long as CSM is okay there is no emergency, but medical follow-up is important.

DIGIT DISLOCATIONS: FINGER AND TOES

Joints in the fingers usually dislocate due to an indirect force that levers the bone ends apart. Active range of motion is impossible, and there is often some degree of CSM impairment. These dislocations often have an associated small avulsion fracture that does not inhibit treatment. Like all dislocations, swelling, pain, and damage from ischemia will increase with time.

TREATMENT OF DIGIT DISLOCATION

Digits usually dislocate at the proximal and distal interphalangeal joints. Reduction is relatively easy. Dislocations of the metacarpal-phalangeal joints (MCP), where the fingers join the hand can be more difficult. Sometimes the base of the phalanx pokes through the joint capsule and becomes trapped there, preventing field reduction. If several attempts fail, splinting and evacuation for surgical reduction is indicated.

Reduction will be easiest right after the injury has occurred, before the swelling and pain gets worse. Grasp the end of the dislocated finger with one hand, and the rest of the finger in the other. Slowly but firmly pull the end of the finger in the direction it is pointing and then, while maintaining traction, swing it back into normal position. You will probably need to wrap the end of your patient's finger in gauze or a bandanna to help keep your grip. Some crepitus will be felt during manipulation.

After manipulation, test passive range of motion to be sure that reduction was successful. The joint will likely be a little swollen and sore with reduced active range of motion. Splint the joint in the mid range, or by padding and taping the finger to the one adjacent (buddy taping). Remember to check CSM before and after reduction. Things should improve with your treatment. Medical follow up should occur within a week, if possible.

DIFFICULT DISLOCATIONS

In the back country, any dislocation that resists your efforts at reduction can become a serious problem. Pain may be severe, and the potential for tissue damage due to ischemia increases with time. If CSM is significantly impaired and cannot be restored by traction and repositioning, immediate evacuation to medical care is warranted.

Some common dislocations should not be reduced in the field. Hip dislocations are difficult to distinguish from hip or pelvis fractures. Pulling on a deformed or immobile hip could lead to catastrophic bleeding. Elbow dislocations are notoriously difficult to reduce. Even when performed successfully, there is a high incidence of complications. Manipulation of either should be performed only in an attempt to restore distal circulation in an ischemic limb.

Digit Dislocation

Reduction:
- TIP to normal anatomy
- Check ROM and distal CSM

Long-Term care:
- RICE and splint or buddy tape to next digit
- Medical follow-up, non-emergent if CSM is OK

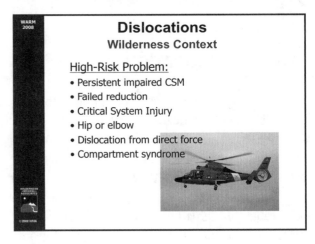

Dislocations
Wilderness Context

High-Risk Problem:
- Persistent impaired CSM
- Failed reduction
- Critical System Injury
- Hip or elbow
- Dislocation from direct force
- Compartment syndrome

Wounds and Burns

15

STRUCTURE AND FUNCTION

The skin is the largest of the body's organs. It performs the remarkable function of protecting your sterile and sensitive internal organs from the flora, fauna, heat, and chill of the wild outdoors. It is also a major component of the thermoregulatory system.

The skin is composed of several layers, the outermost being the epidermis. The outer surface of the epidermis is called the *statum corneum*, which is actually a layer of dead skin cells and bacteria. These cells are continuously being generated and shed at an impressive rate—some 50 million per day. This process, similar to the continuous flow of mucous from the respiratory system, is part of how we protect ourselves from the billions of microbes with which we share our existence.

The dermis is the next layer, and contains larger blood vessels, sweat glands, hair follicles, and most of the nerve endings of the skin. Sweat and oil excreted onto the skin surface help with protection by killing some bacteria and reinforcing the skin's barrier effect. The total thickness of the dermal layer varies from a half a millimeter on the eyelids to three or four millimeters on the palms and soles.

The blood vessels in the dermis are capable of a dramatic change in volume as they constrict or dilate for thermoregulation or the need to maintain core perfusion pressure. When fully vasodilated, the skin can hold up to three liters of blood; when fully vasoconstricted, as in severe shell/core effect, the skin may retain as little as 30 milliliters of blood.

Under the dermis is a layer of fat. In some places, like the buttocks or belly, this layer can be many centimeters thick. In other locations, like the back of the hand, it may be only a few cells thick. Below the fat lies a layer of tough connective tissue called *fascia*. This is typically shiny-white and fibrous in appearance, and covers underlying muscle, bone, organs, and joints.

Problems begin when the protective outer layer of skin is damaged and the soft tissue beneath is exposed. This allows bacteria and viruses to invade unprotected tissue and lets body fluids escape. Deep wounds where the fascia is interrupted are at high-risk for infection. Extensive soft tissue injury can cause shock and hypothermia.

All wounds damage blood vessels and cause bleeding. The body attempts to control blood loss by automatically constricting blood vessels at the injury site. Chemical components called *clotting factors* interact with platelets in the blood to form a blood clot. Under most circumstances, bleeding will stop

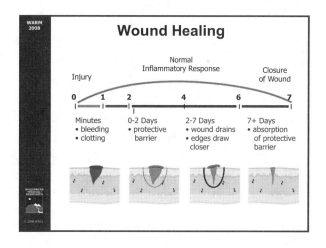

within 15 minutes. Sometimes it needs a little help in the form of direct pressure or other bleeding control techniques.

After the blood loss has been stopped, the slower process of wound repair begins. The initial stages of natural wound cleansing occur over a period of several days. The clot surface dries, forming a natural bandage in the form of a scab. Underlying tissue is further protected by the process of inflammation that provides a protective barrier beneath the injury.

Contaminants like dirt and bacteria are flushed out as the wound drains. By the third or fourth day, the protective barriers are established and cleansing is well underway. Redness, warmth, swelling, and pain begin to decrease as the normal inflammatory response subsides.

After six to ten days, the wound is very resistant to contamination. Wound edges migrate together as the collagen fibers within the clot contract. Scar formation and complete healing continue over the next six to twelve months.

WOUND ASSESSMENT

There are many terms such as laceration, avulsion, and abrasion used to describe wounds. But, for field purposes, wounds can be assessed generically as simple or high risk. This is analogous to the stable or unstable assessment of musculoskeletal trauma. Simple wounds offer no risk of life-threatening bleeding and do not represent a significant risk of infection. They can be managed in the field, with evacuation to medical care as convenient.

Simple wounds may involve the dermis and subcutaneous fat, but they do not penetrate the fascia. There is no contamination of muscle, bone, tendons, or joint structure. Simple wounds are clean and free of devitalized or macerated tissue. A superficial cut from a clean knife is an example.

Some wounds have the potential to cause cosmetic or functional defects as they heal. Examples include wounds of the face, hands, and genitalia. You may

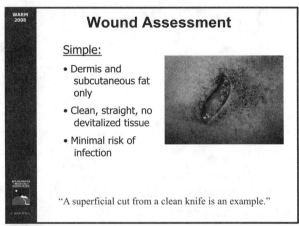

Wound Assessment

Simple:

- Dermis and subcutaneous fat only
- Clean, straight, no devitalized tissue
- Minimal risk of infection

"A superficial cut from a clean knife is an example."

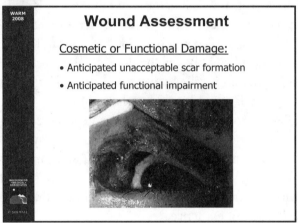

Wound Assessment

Cosmetic or Functional Damage:

- Anticipated unacceptable scar formation
- Anticipated functional impairment

choose to refer these wounds for immediate care when the risk of evacuation is low. The best results will be obtained when wound repair is accomplished within several hours, but acceptable wound repair can be accomplished days later, if necessary.

HIGH-RISK WOUNDS

High-risk wounds are those that carry a significant risk of infection or are likely to cause functional problems during early healing. Also labeled as high-risk are wounds associated with life-threatening bleeding or critical system injury. Aggressive field treatment and early evacuation for debridement is ideal.

Grossly Contaminated: Injuries with imbedded foreign material, such as gravel, sawdust, or clothing fibers, harbor bacteria that is difficult to dislodge.

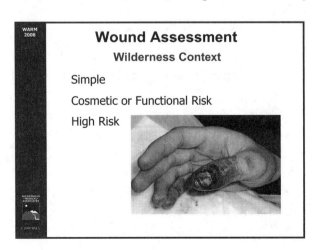

Wound Assessment

Wilderness Context

Simple

Cosmetic or Functional Risk

High Risk

Mangled: Wounds that involve crushed, shredded, or dead tissue provide growth medium for bacteria.

Deep: Wounds that penetrate the fascia to expose joints, tendons, and bones are difficult to clean adequately and prone to serious infection.

Bites (from humans or other animals): Mouths harbor a wide variety of virulent bugs. Human bites are among the worst. Cats are pretty bad, too. Any wound exposed to human or animal salvia constitutes a bite wound.

Punctures: A small opening in the skin with a wound track that extends through several layers of tissue deposits bacteria in areas that are unable to drain properly.

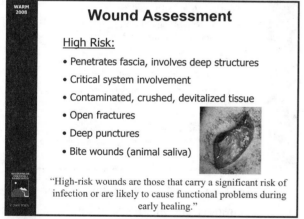

Wound Assessment

High Risk:

• Penetrates fascia, involves deep structures

• Critical system involvement

• Contaminated, crushed, devitalized tissue

• Open fractures

• Deep punctures

• Bite wounds (animal saliva)

"High-risk wounds are those that carry a significant risk of infection or are likely to cause functional problems during early healing."

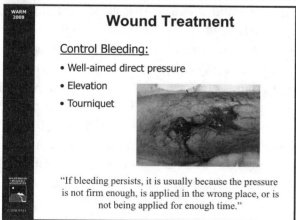

Wound Treatment

Control Bleeding:

• Well-aimed direct pressure

• Elevation

• Tourniquet

"If bleeding persists, it is usually because the pressure is not firm enough, is applied in the wrong place, or is not being applied for enough time."

Wound assessment is an important skill for the wilderness medical practitioner. Some wounds can appear simple, involving only the dermis and fat layers.

On closer inspection, you may find that the fascia is interrupted and deep structures are contaminated. A good field examination may take some time and involve careful probing with instruments or fingers.

The fascia is easily identified as a tough, dull-white layer of tissue resembling unfinished fiberglass. Underlying structures like tendon, bone, and joint surface appear shiny and white or yellow. Muscle underlying the fascia appears deep red, like a raw steak.

The depth of the wound in millimeters is far less significant than the layers penetrated. An eyelid laceration a few millimeters deep may be high-risk, while a wound on the buttocks several centimeters deep is considered simple. Puncture wounds often appear very benign on the surface, but carry a substantial risk of infection to deep structures. Avulsion flaps should be lifted and inspected for debris, and probed for deep structure involvement.

Wounds to the chest or abdomen may enter the organ cavities. There will sometimes be an obvious hollow space, visible or probed. These are very serious and often involve critical system injury. Emergency evacuation to surgical care is lifesaving.

Remember that open wounds also present risk to the examiner. Don't forget to protect your eyes, skin, and mucous membranes from contact with blood and exudates. Wear gloves, eye protection, and keep your mouth shut or wear a mask.

FIELD TREATMENT OF WOUNDS

The initial field treatment of both simple and high-risk wounds is the same. Stop the bleeding, inspect and clean, and dress and monitor for infection. Evacuation should be initiated for high-risk wounds.

An impaled object is best removed by a surgeon in a hospital, but evacuating a patient with an impaled object will often risk more tissue damage than pulling it out. As long as the object remains imbedded in the tissue, infection is inevitable. In most cases, impaled objects should be removed in the field and the wounds cleaned like any other. But, if it is clear that you are going to do significant damage trying to

See erratum in front cover

remove the object, stabilize it in place and evacuate as quickly and carefully as you can. Never remove an impaled object from the globe of the eye because

---

WARM 2008

Wound Treatment
WILDERNESS PROTOCOL

Remove Impaled Objects Unless:

- Impaled in the globe of the eye
- Removal will cause significant problems:
  - tissue destruction
  - severe bleeding
  - unmanageable pain

© 2008 WMA

---

the fluid inside the eye cannot be replaced and any amount lost will doom the patient's vision.

Bleeding is best controlled with direct pressure and will usually stop within 15 minutes as the clotting mechanism is activated. If bleeding persists, it is usually because the pressure is not firm enough, is applied in the wrong place, or is not being applied for enough time. Elevation of an injured extremity can also help reduce bleeding by reducing the blood pressure in the effected extremity. Ice will help constrict blood vessels in the area of the injury.

A tourniquet may be used temporarily to slow major bleeding while you find the bleeding site or in cases where you are too busy managing other critical system problems. A tourniquet can also be used for short periods to allow for adequate visualization for wound cleaning. It is a very useful tool and is only dangerous when left in place long enough to cause ischemia to infarction.

A proper tourniquet is composed of a wide, soft band applied just proximal to the injury. Enough pressure must be applied to stop arterial blood flow, or venous congestion and edema will develop. As long as there is no risk of frostbite, a tourniquet can be left in place for up to an hour.

Long-term management of any wound requires early wound cleaning to help prevent infection. The use of prophylactic antibiotics is limited in the

civilized setting, but should be considered for the wilderness context due to the greater difficulties involved in wound care. The initial dose should be

---

WARM 2008

Wound Treatment
WILDERNESS PROTOCOL

Inspect and Clean:

- Clean surrounding skin surface.
- Irrigate with copious amounts of clean water or 1% PI solution.
- Explore wound and remove foreign bodies.
- Cut away dead tissue.

"Proper wound cleaning can take quite a bit of time. Make yourself and your patient comfortable and do a thorough job."

WARM 2008

Wound Treatment
WILDERNESS PROTOCOL

High-Risk Wound Care:

- Clean as with any other wound unless there is risk of life-threatening bleeding
- Early evacuation
- Consider antibiotics if authorized
- Contact local health department about rabies risk in mammal bites

"Gentle probing…may reveal a previously unnoticed laceration of the fascia exposing muscle or joint space to contamination."

---

supplies are limited, using a 1% solution of povidone iodine may reduce the incidence of infection. There is no significant advantage to using sterile saline.

There is an advantage, however, to applying a little pressure to the irrigation stream. Studies demonstrate that the ideal irrigation pressure is between four and eight pounds per square inch. You won't be able to measure that in the field, of course, but it can be approximated with a steady stream from a 30–60 cc syringe and an 18 gauge catheter. You are not trying to sterilize the wound, just flushing out debris and reducing the bacteria count to levels which can be managed by the body's immune system.

It is harmful to irrigate a wound with full strength iodine preparations (typically 10%) or hydrogen peroxide. Iodine and peroxide kill both bacteria and body cells, leaving a partially sterilized wound lined with dead tissue. This can actually increase the risk of infection. Use only clean water or saline, a 1% iodine solution, or a product specifically formulated for use in open wounds. It is interesting to note that soaking a wound in a basin of saline or iodine as is often practiced in clinics and hospitals may actually increase the risk of infection.

Continue cleaning by removing any imbedded debris that was not flushed out by irrigation. A toothbrush, forceps, scissors, and a head-lamp are useful tools for this. Cut away any dead tissue or loose fat. These are likely to become a site for bacterial growth.

Proper wound cleaning can take quite a bit of time. Make yourself and your patient comfortable and do a thorough job. It may be inconvenient, but it will save you a lot of time and trouble by preventing an infection.

Once cleaned, the wound should be carefully inspected to determine the extent and depth of the defect. Gentle probing with a sterilized instrument or gloved finger may reveal a previously unnoticed laceration of the fascia exposing muscle or joint space to contamination. Treatment and evacuation for high-risk wound care would then be a priority.

In most cases, the wound is then covered with a

or offshore setting, the risk of wound closure usually far outweighs the benefit. Early wound cleaning is essential, early wound closure is not. Wound repair or scar revision can be safely delayed for days or weeks if necessary.

The exception would be simple wounds that do not penetrate the full thickness of the dermis. These may safely be closed after cleaning. This is mostly a matter of convenience. Steri-strips, butterflies, and wound closure glue are equally effective but will require protection from moisture and contamination. Temporary wound closure with tape might also be indicated for functional reasons, such on the hand for paddling and feet for hiking. This type of functional taping should be removed at the end of the day.

BANDAGES AND DRESSINGS FOR A HOSTILE ENVIRONMENT

The combination of bandage and dressing should allow for wound drainage while preventing contamination. The goal of long-term wound care is to preserve and enhance oxygenation and perfusion of the tissue, and prevent infection. Prolonged shell/core effect or local vasoconstriction of the hands and feet in wet and cold conditions are typical impediments

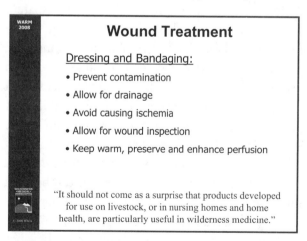

Wound Closure
Wilderness Context

- The desire or need for wound repair with sutures or staples does not warrant a high-risk evacuation.
- Acceptable closure may be performed by a medical professional days later.
- Wound closure in the field can increase the risk of infection.

"Early wound cleaning is essential, early closure is not."

Wound Treatment

Dressing and Bandaging:
- Prevent contamination
- Allow for drainage
- Avoid causing ischemia
- Allow for wound inspection
- Keep warm, preserve and enhance perfusion

"It should not come as a surprise that products developed for use on livestock, or in nursing homes and home health, are particularly useful in wilderness medicine."

sterile dressing to prevent outside contamination and to absorb wound drainage. Allowing for drainage is important to normal healing. Wound closure with tape, sutures, staples, or glue can create an obstructed hollow space prone to infection. In the backcountry

to healing. Altitude is also a problem. Wound healing is significantly delayed at 3000 meters, and almost impossible above 6000 meters.

High-risk wounds with exposed soft tissue, bone, or other deep structures are best dressed with a wet,

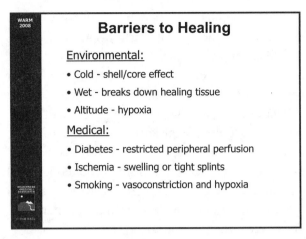

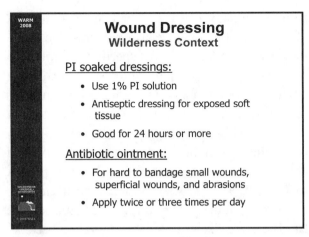

anti-bacterial surface next to the wound. Drying will further damage tissue. Covered xeroform or silver impregnated dressings are ideal, but a dressing soaked with dilute povidone iodine solution will suffice.

The surface in contact with the open wound should begin sterile, and remain that way for as long as possible. The bandage should not impair circulation or prevent wound examination. Meeting these criteria on a wet and dirty expedition or evacuation can be quite a challenge. Typical first-aid kit adhesive tape and white roller gauze perform poorly in the backcountry or marine environment.

Newer dressings designed for long-term care of open wounds offer medical practitioners some good options for backcountry use. A sterile, transparent semi-permeable membrane can be left in place for several days. Semi-permeable membranes are also combined with colloidal dressings to absorb exudates, keep the wound moist, and prevent external contamination even in very wet and dirty situations. The dressings are expensive, but far superior to the standard-issue first aid supplies.

An inexpensive roller bandage known as *vet wrap*, originally developed for veterinary use, can be used for splints or to hold dressings in place far more effectively than tape or an elastic bandage. It is water resistant, self amalgamating, and reusable. Abrasions and shallow wounds in which only the superficial layers of skin is affected can be dressed with antibiotic ointment alone or with an easily removed sterile dressing. Since the most common anticipated problem with abrasions is infection, frequent cleaning

and inspection is a priority. Antibiotic ointment can also be used alone in difficult-to-bandage places like eyelids and ears.

Wounds over or involving joints should be splinted if conditions and travel allow. High-risk wounds should receive early medical attention whenever possible, especially where open fracture is suspected. Your ideal evacuation plan would have your patient out of the woods within 48 hours. During your walk out, the wound should receive the same careful attention as any other. This is especially true for the removal of debris and irrigation. If your treatment is particularly effective, infection may never start.

A tetanus vaccine booster should be given to anyone with an open wound who has not had a vaccination within ten years, or five years for high-risk wounds. This is best done within 24 hours of injury. You can keep this from becoming a problem by keeping your routine tetanus vaccinations up to date, and ensuring that everyone else in your group does the same.

Monitor the wound for signs of infection whether or not you choose to evacuate. You should also monitor the CSM distal to the injury as you would with a musculoskeletal problem. Bandages, splints, and swelling can create ischemia here as well.

EVISCERATION

Internal organs protruding from a wound is a gruesome scenario, but certainly possible with penetrating trauma to the abdomen or thorax. Eviscerated organs should be covered with wet gauze or occlusive dressings like plastic wrap, and the patient evacuated to surgical care as rapidly as possible. Allowing a bent-knee position in the litter will reduce the tension of the abdominal wall and help prevent ischemia. Although positioning the patient for transport may result in spontaneous reduction of the evisceration, no attempt should be made in the field to push organs back into the body cavity. Shock, hypothermia, and systemic infection are anticipated problems.

TRAUMATIC AMPUTATION

Full or incomplete amputations should be treated with the expectation that replantation is possible, or at least that tissue and skin from the amputated part can be useful in repair of the stump. Successful replantation has been accomplished after as much as 24 hours of ischemia. The surgeon should decide which injuries are candidates for replantation; your job is to get your patient and the amputated part to the appropriate facility as soon as possible.

The ideal field treatment is to wrap the amputated part in a gauze sponge soaked with saline, place it in a plastic bag, and float the bag in ice water. Bleeding from the patient's amputation site should be controlled only with direct pressure, and the wound maintained with moist dressings. Tourniquets and clamps should be used only if bleeding cannot be otherwise controlled.

In the absence of ice and sterile saline, a dressing moistened in clean water or 1% PI solution will suffice. Keep the part as cool as possible without freezing and continue with the evacuation. Partially amputated extremities are treated the same way while still attached to the patient. Do not cut the part free.

If managed correctly, an amputated extremity is not a life-threatening injury. In spite of the drama and urgency of the situation, do not risk the lives of the patient and rescuers to preserve the possibility of replantation. A live patient with an artificial limb confirms a successful rescue. A fatality during the evacuation does not.

RABIES

Rabies is a viral infection and nearly always fatal in humans. It is transmitted via the saliva of an infected animal, usually by biting. It is most common in bats, dogs and cats, and mesopredators like raccoons, fox, and skunks. Most of the time, an exposure is obvious. With bats, a bite may go unnoticed. The mere presence of a bat inside a house may be reason enough to give rabies post-exposure prophylaxis to the human inhabitants.

Post-exposure prophylaxis (PEP) consists of immediate and vigorous wound cleaning with warm water and soap, followed by irrigation with povidone iodine solution. In animal bite wounds, the benefit of killing a potentially fatal virus justifies the risk of tissue damage caused by the soap or solution. The patient should then be urgently transferred to a medical facility equipped to provide rabies immune globulin and vaccine.

WOUND INFECTION

In normal wound healing, the pain, swelling, redness, and inflammation will decrease quickly within the first two or three days. If the wound becomes infected, these signs and symptoms will begin to increase instead. Pus develops as the cellular debris and edema fluid accumulates in the wound. Infection is a possibility in any wound at any time during the healing process, but is most likely to develop within two to four days after injury.

WARM 2008
Traumatic Amputation
• Wrap the part in sterile, moist, dressing
• Keep the part cool, transport with patient
• Control bleeding with direct pressure or tourniquet
• Do not complete partial amputations
• Splint the extremity
• Emergency evacuation

If a local infection spreads, it will ultimately enter the general circulation and cause a systemic infection. This is referred to as blood poisoning, lymphangitis, or sepsis. The symptoms of this whole-body inflammation include fever, skin redness, body aches, general malaise, and ultimately septic shock (a form of vascular shock). Even simple wounds like blisters that become infected present some risk of progressing to life-threatening sepsis.

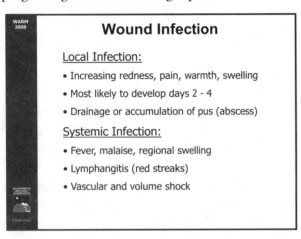

TREATMENT OF WOUND INFECTION

If the infected wound has been closed with tape, sutures, or staples it should be opened, irrigated, and allowed to drain. Avoid forcefully squeezing the purulent material from the wound or you may drive bacteria through the protective barrier into healthy tissues. At some point in your past, you've probably seen a minor pimple become a big abscess as a result of this practice.

If an abscess has formed in the dermis close to the

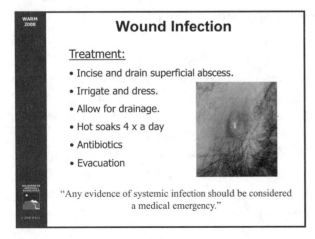

surface, it can be safely opened with a sharp knife, irrigated, and allowed to drain. Clean the skin surface with antiseptic or soap and knick the pus pocket with a sterile blade. This procedure is reserved for those cases where the pus pocket is obvious and superficial. Don't attempt to incise anything in the deeper layers of the skin or soft tissue.

Applying heat to the infected area will increase circulation and help the body fight the infection locally. Use as much heat as your patient can comfortably tolerate against normal skin for 30 minutes at a time, as often as five to six times a day. Heat can be applied in the form of hot soaks or contact with a warm rock or hot water bottle.

Drainage and heat applications will often cure a wound infection, but antibiotics are considered to be part of the ideal treatment where surgical care is unavailable. Although not usually within the scope of practice for first responders and EMTs in the urban context, these drugs may be a worthy addition to your wilderness treatment protocols. If your duties take you days away from medical help, consider obtaining formal authorization and instructions from a medical practitioner.

Although the routine use of prophylactic antibiotics is controversial and often of limited benefit, it should be considered for high-risk wounds in settings where surgical follow-up may be delayed for days or weeks. Deep punctures and open fractures are good examples. Antibiotics must be administered within an hour or two of injury to be effective in prophylaxis.

Any evidence of systemic infection should be considered a medical emergency. Broad-spectrum antibiotics should be started immediately. Some oral medications can be just as effective as those given by injection, and easily used by Wilderness First Responders and EMTs with the proper authorization. Urgent evacuation is required. Septic shock is an anticipated problem.

BURNS

For field management, we need to know the depth and extent of burns, as well as location. The extent is described in terms of body surface area (BSA), and critical locations include hands, feet, genitalia, and the respiratory system. The circulatory system can also be affected because burns can cause rapid fluid loss resulting in shock. Hypothermia is an anticipated problem in large burns.

Estimates of irregular burns can be made using the size of the patient's palm, which is about 1% of the body surface area. The depth of burn refers to how deep the damage goes. This can be difficult to estimate, particularly where different areas are burned to different depths.

In superficial (first degree) burns, skin integrity is not disrupted. Capillaries and nerves are intact.

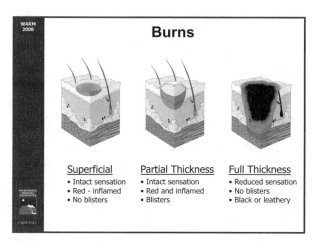

Inflammation occurs with redness, pain, and warmth. This is your typical sunburn.

In partial-thickness (second degree) burns, the skin surface is damaged, but the injury is limited to outer layers. These are characterized by intact and denuded blisters and reddened or pink skin. Surface capillaries are damaged, but deeper skin blood vessels and nerves are intact. There is fluid loss, redness, warmth, and pain.

Full-thickness (third degree) burns penetrate the dermis to involve the subcutaneous soft tissues. Skin blood vessels and nerves are destroyed. The burned area may appear charred black, or gray. The area may not be painful due to loss of nerve endings. Normal inflammation cannot occur, and as a result, blisters do not develop. Small full-thickness burns may appear to be less serious because of this.

As with other injuries, look first for potentially life-threatening problems. These will usually come in the form of volume shock or respiratory distress. High-risk burns are those that include anticipated major problems with critical body systems, severe pain, infection, or scar formation.

HIGH-RISK BURNS

The following signs and symptoms should motivate careful monitoring and early evacuation to definitive medical care, preferably in a burn center.

> ***Any respiratory system involvement***: Burned respiratory passages will develop the same inflammation, blisters, and fluid loss that are seen on the skin. Signs and symptoms include singed facial hair, burned lips, sooty sputum, and persistent cough. Respiratory distress may develop from pulmonary edema or from swelling and obstruction in the airways. It can develop quickly or slowly over a period of hours. Respiratory burns carry a mortality rate of about 20%.
>
> ***Partial-thickness burns of the face, genitalia, and hands***: Any significant burns in these areas can cause problems with swelling and ischemia in the short term; and mobility and scarring in the long-term.
>
> ***Circumferential burns***: Burns that completely circle an extremity can cause distal ischemia as swelling develops.
>
> ***Burns of any degree greater than 10% BSA***: Large burns carry the anticipated problem of volume shock and hypothermia. Any full-thickness burn: Any full-thickness burn is at high-risk for infection.
>
> ***Chemical burns***: It can be difficult to fully arrest the burning process as some chemicals react with the skin. Damage can continue for hours afterward.
>
> ***Electrical burns***: Skin damage may be minor, but man-made electrical current can cause extensive injury to internal organs

and tissues. Lightning tends to cause only superficial burns and little internal electrical injury.

Burns of very young or very old patients: Infants and the elderly have a more difficult time compensating for injury.

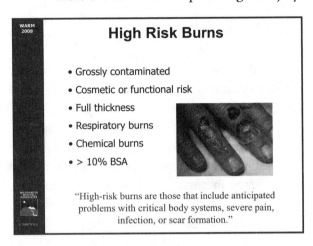

High Risk Burns

- Grossly contaminated
- Cosmetic or functional risk
- Full thickness
- Respiratory burns
- Chemical burns
- > 10% BSA

"High-risk burns are those that include anticipated problems with critical body systems, severe pain, infection, or scar formation."

TREATMENT OF BURNS

The initial treatment for burns is to remove the heat energy. The fastest way to do this is to immerse the patient or injured part in water. Fortunately, this is almost instinctive as it serves to relieve pain as well. If the burn is greater than about 10% BSA, limit your cooling to prevent hypothermia. For most chemical burns, continued irrigation with water will not only cool the area, but help remove the chemical itself. Irrigation of chemical burns should continue for at least 30 minutes.

If the burn is not a life-threatening emergency,

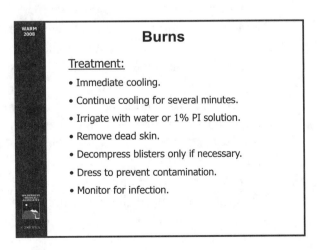

Burns

Treatment:

- Immediate cooling.
- Continue cooling for several minutes.
- Irrigate with water or 1% PI solution.
- Remove dead skin.
- Decompress blisters only if necessary.
- Dress to prevent contamination.
- Monitor for infection.

clean and dress it with antibiotic dressings like a minor abrasion or use one of the long-term wound care products. This can be done along with the application of cool soaks for pain relief. Monitor for infection as you would with any open wound.

If the burn falls under the category of high-risk,

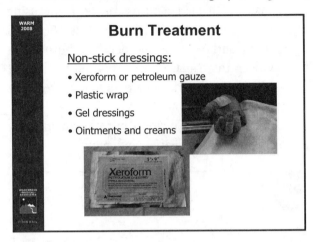

Burn Treatment

Non-stick dressings:

- Xeroform or petroleum gauze
- Plastic wrap
- Gel dressings
- Ointments and creams

plan to have the patient to medical care within about 48 hours if possible. If the burn involves significant damage to the respiratory or circulatory system, emergency evacuation should be initiated with early access to ALS. Ideally, transport directly to a burn center.

In a wilderness setting, even a sunburn can be a significant problem in if it occupies a large area of skin surface. Ultraviolet radiation causes inflammation of the dermis and epidermis, inhibiting skin function and causing pain and redness. You should anticipate all of the same problems inherent in any large surface area burn: volume shock, thermoregulatory problems, pain, and infection.

Dressing a large surface area burn can be difficult. The goal is to minimize contamination and reduce evaporative cooling. An improvised dressing can consist of a clean cotton tee-shirt covered with a waterproof clothing layer. Plastic kitchen wrap will also work. Immediate attention should be given to maintaining hydration and body core temperature. The patient will need food, fluids, and protection during evacuation. Prophylactic antibiotics may be indicated for large or contaminated burns. Aloe vera gel is useful to relieve pain and provide some topical antibiotic and anti-inflammatory effect.

BLISTERS

Blisters, like the kind you get on your heel while hiking, are caused by the heat generated by your boots and socks rubbing against your skin. The damage results in swelling and inflammation. Although a blister is only a superficial wound, it can become a major transportation problem.

Blisters progress through three stages beginning with a *hot spot*, progressing to a partial-thickness burn, and then breaking to become a contaminated superficial wound. The stage at which you confront blisters and your logistical situation will determine your treatment. Generally, they are treated just like other partial-thickness burns.

TREATMENT OF BLISTERS

If you can stop the friction, you can prevent a blister from forming. Advise your patient to change her socks, adjust her laces, and cover the sore area with a liner sock, smooth surface tape, gel dressings or mole skin. You can also apply antibiotic ointment to lubricate the area and reduce friction.

If a blister does form, it is important to remember that a blister is a sterile wound until it breaks. The best treatment is to leave the overlying skin intact until healing can start. Small blisters can be covered with gel dressing. Larger ones will usually cause some degree of disability unless you can take the pressure off.

If the blister has formed in a bad spot, like the back of the heel, you may have to drain it to allow the patient to keep moving. Like draining an abscess, clean the skin around and over the blister with soap and water or antiseptic. Sterilize a sharp knife blade by flame or iodine. Make a small V-cut in the blister at the lower margin and allow the fluid to drain out. Leave the skin over the blister intact to act as its own sterile dressing. Cover the area with antibiotic ointment and dress it as you might a hot spot. Like any open wound, it must be cleaned and dressed daily and monitored for signs of infection. Avoid draining blood-filled blisters.

Open blisters occur when a blister has broken into a non-sterile environment. It should be treated like an abrasion. Cut away the dead skin and irrigate to remove debris and cover the wound with antibiotic ointment and sterile dressings. Clean daily and monitor for infection. Fix the source of friction with padding or tape.

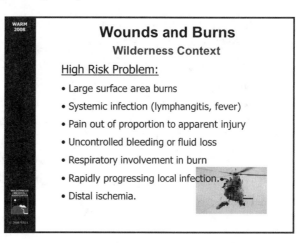

WARM 2008	**Wounds and Burns**
	Wilderness Context

High Risk Problem:
• Large surface area burns
• Systemic infection (lymphangitis, fever)
• Pain out of proportion to apparent injury
• Uncontrolled bleeding or fluid loss
• Respiratory involvement in burn
• Rapidly progressing local infection.
• Distal ischemia.

Blisters

Prevent Friction and Heat:
• Moleskin, donut dressing
• Smooth tape
• Gel dressings

Treatment:
• Unroof blister if it appears infected.
• Drain blister if it prevents travel.
• Dress as partial thickness burn.

CASE STUDY: WOUNDS

Scene: Fishing vessel in the Gulf Stream approximately 300 miles SE of Cape Cod. The weather was mild, but expected to deteriorate over the next 24 hours.

S: A 43-year-old crewmen on a fishing vessel was struck on the head by a swinging davit when a long-line parted. He was found sitting on deck with a large and freely bleeding laceration across the top of his head. He remembered everything about the event. He denied neck pain, and has no other complaints. He denied allergies, was taking no medications, was well fed and warm, had no significant medical history, and was up to date on his tetanus vaccination.

O: Awake, oriented, and cooperative man holding a blood-soaked kerchief on his head. Blood covered his left shoulder and chest, and there was a large pool on the deck He has no neck deformity or tenderness, has full range of motion, and has normal sensation of extremities with no numbness or tingling. The scalp has a four cm laceration, clean and straight, through the skin and subcutaneous tissue to the skull. No depression or bone fragments can be seen or felt. Vital Signs at 18:05 were—BP: 112/78, P: 88, R: 16, C: Awake and oriented, T: normal, Skin: normal color and temperature.

A: 1. Scalp wound
         A': Wound infection (unlikely)

P: Direct pressure to stop bleeding. Clean surrounding scalp and hair with soap and water. Irrigate the wound with water. Dress with sterile dressings and a hat to hold them in place. Monitor and redress at least daily. Follow up with physician in Bermuda during the planned port call in 3 days.

Discussion: The scalp did just what it was designed to do. By slipping and tearing, it absorbed enough of the force of the impact to protect the skull and brain. There was no head injury, just a scalp wound. As is common to the scalp, bleeding was profuse but easily controlled with direct pressure. Although it looked like a lot of blood, vital signs show that not enough was lost to produce shock. Because of the rich blood supply, even deep scalp wounds usually heal well with a very low incidence of infection. There was no emergency here.

Section IV

Environmental Medicine

Thermoregulation

16

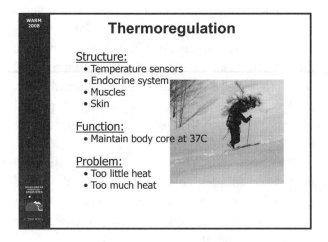

Thermoregulation

Structure:
- Temperature sensors
- Endocrine system
- Muscles
- Skin

Function:
- Maintain body core at 37C

Problem:
- Too little heat
- Too much heat

STRUCTURE AND FUNCTION

The core of the human body operates most efficiently at or very near a temperature of 37° C. The brain adjusts heat production and retention automatically based on information from temperature sensors in the skin and body core. This thermoregulatory system uses muscles to generate heat, the skin to dissipate heat, and the endocrine system to control metabolism. Blood vessels in the skin dilate or constrict to dissipate or preserve heat. Sweat glands release fluid to enhance cooling by evaporation. Shivering produces heat with involuntary exercise. You can watch this compensation mechanism work, but it is not under your direct control.

Because your body core is always at a temperature of about 37° C, your conscious perception of hot or cold comes from sensors in your skin. When heat energy is released into your skin by contact with a warm object, you feel warmth. When heat energy is removed from your skin, you feel cold. In the healthy individual the perception of being warm or cold, and the need to produce or dissipate heat, is based primarily on conditions affecting the body shell.

A number of things can influence this perception. Alcohol, for example, is a vasodilator that allows more warm blood to perfuse the skin surface, reversing the shell/core compensation. It impairs normal shivering and inhibits effective thermoregulatory sensation and response. When you down a shot of schnapps to stay warm, usually while standing around an ice-fishing hole in the dead of winter, a satisfying feeling of warmth spreads throughout your body as sensors in the skin detect the heat contributed by the surge of blood from the body core. But, you are not actually warming yourself at all. You might feel better, but you are actually losing more heat to the cold night air. If you were to keep drinking you could "warm" yourself right into hypothermia.

This example reminds us that our conscious efforts are important to thermoregulation, too. Even the best body morphology will not keep you healthy if you don't pay attention to hydration, calories and shelter. Problems with heat and cold often have their origins in poor judgment.

Problems with thermoregulation can also develop when the function of the system is impaired by illness, injury, toxins, or medication. The system can also be overwhelmed by environmental extremes. Maintaining the function of the thermoregulatory system is a key element of patient care in the wilderness setting.

HYPOTHERMIA

Cold response is a normal reaction to feeling cold and starts long before the body core temperature begins to fall with the onset of hypothermia. Shell/core compensation reduces heat loss to the environment, while shivering increases heat production from muscle activity. The discomfort you feel by being cold motivates your conscious effort to add layers of clothing and get out of the weather. If the system works normally and is not overwhelmed by an extreme challenge, normal core temperature and mental status is preserved.

Nobody will be able to mount an effective cold response when short on food and fluids. Shivering is a very efficient form of heat production, but requires a tremendous amount of energy. Living outside in a cold environment can require more than 6000 calories a day. Adequate glycogen stores and easily digested food must be available to maintain the effort. Normal body fluid volume is also required to effectively generate and distribute heat.

An anticipated and annoying problem associated with the cold response is cold diuresis. This is the

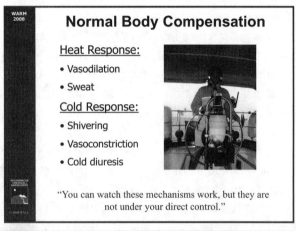

Normal Body Compensation

Heat Response:
• Vasodilation
• Sweat

Cold Response:
• Shivering
• Vasoconstriction
• Cold diuresis

"You can watch these mechanisms work, but they are not under your direct control."

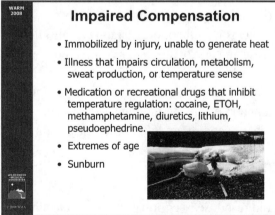

Impaired Compensation

• Immobilized by injury, unable to generate heat
• Illness that impairs circulation, metabolism, sweat production, or temperature sense
• Medication or recreational drugs that inhibit temperature regulation: cocaine, ETOH, methamphetamine, diuretics, lithium, pseudoephedrine.
• Extremes of age
• Sunburn

tendency of the body to produce more urine when shell/core compensation occurs. As blood is shunted from the shell into the core, the kidneys sense an increase in fluid volume in the central circulation and act to get rid of some of it. Cold diuresis and the logistics involved in obtaining fresh water in an extreme environment can lead to dehydration.

Although cold response is normal and healthy, it carries the anticipated problem of hypothermia. A number of factors can accelerate the process. A patient who is immobilized by injury will not be able to exercise or consciously act to retain heat. Drugs that cause vasodilatation of the skin will result in greater heat loss. Chronic endocrine system problems like hypothyroidism or diabetes can inhibit the body's ability to sense or respond to temperature changes. Elderly people have less muscle mass and a reduced ability to perceive and respond to heat loss. Children tend to have less body fat and a greater surface area to mass ratio which will also increase the rate of heat loss.

Reversing cold response requires insulation, protection, calories, and fluids. To do this most effectively, you need to understand the physics of heat production, retention, and dissipation. Fortunately, it is not too complicated.

Heat energy flows from warmer objects like your patient to colder objects like the ground or litter. The mechanisms are *conduction*, *convection*, *evaporation*, and *radiation*. In protecting and packaging your patient, you must consider all of these forms of heat loss:

> ***Conduction*** is heat transfer between objects in contact. The more dense the object, the faster heat energy will be transferred. Your patient will lose heat much more quickly to the cold, hard ground he is laying on than the low-density foam pad that you should have placed under him.

> ***Convection*** is heat transfer via moving fluids, including air and water. Although air is the least dense substance, there is an infinite supply of it. Heat lost to wind or even to the air billowing in and out of loose clothing can be considerable. Water works the same way, just 25 times faster.

> ***Evaporation*** refers to the heat energy absorbed by water as it turns into water

vapor. The body uses this very efficient mechanism for cooling in the form of sweat. Water evaporating from the skin will cool your patient very efficiently whether he needs it or not.

Radiant heat energy is emitted and absorbed by all objects, including your patient. This is long-wave electromagnetic radiation well below the frequency of visible light. This energy is the warmth you feel from sunlight or a campfire. Radiant heat from your body can be absorbed by dense or thick clothing, or reflected back to you by a foil covering.

Non-compressible insulation such as a closed-cell foam pad should be used to protect the patient from conductive heat loss to the ground or other cold objects. High-loft, low-density insulation such as a synthetic or down sleeping bag forms a dead air space around the patient, reducing convective heat loss and trapping the radiant heat being emitted by the patient. A waterproof *vapor barrier* around the insulation prevents wetting of the package from rain or snow and reduces the evaporative cooling from moisture already on the patient.

Support for heat production is equally critical. Your patient needs calories and fluids to fuel shivering. Simple sugars are best at first. They will be quickly absorbed and converted into energy. Complex carbohydrates, fats, and protein can be added later to maintain heat production.

Adding heat in the form of warm liquids or heat packs is comforting, but not as useful as the calories, hydration, and exercise. The heat energy in a cup of hot tea is minimal compared to the heat that will be produced when the patient burns the four tablespoons of honey you put into it. Don't delay food and fluids while waiting for your stove to heat up.

Most of the time, your efforts will be successful. Sometimes, the system fails or is overwhelmed by environmental conditions resulting in a drop in body core temperature. Shell/core compensation persists, shivering continues, and your patient's mental status begins to decay. Your anticipated problem has become the existing problem.

MILD HYPOTHERMIA

Rescuers will certainly think of hypothermia in cases of obvious and extreme exposure such as cold-water immersion. Even dressed for cold weather, ice water can kill you within an hour. Nobody will miss the diagnosis in situations like this.

However, in most backcountry situations the onset of hypothermia is insidious more often than dramatic. It progresses slowly and quietly in a patient who is just a little cold for a long time. In this case, the problem is easy to overlook.

Hypothermia may be the primary problem you are treating or a side effect of environmental conditions. It is a common complication in trauma cases where a patient has remained immobile for hours while

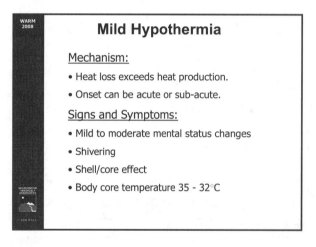

Mild Hypothermia

Mechanism:
• Heat loss exceeds heat production.
• Onset can be acute or sub-acute.

Signs and Symptoms:
• Mild to moderate mental status changes
• Shivering
• Shell/core effect
• Body core temperature 35 - 32°C

waiting for rescue. It also develops in rescue team members waiting for hours for instructions.

In rapid onset cases like cold water immersion, there is often a radical difference in temperature between the cold body shell and the still relatively warm body core. Generally, the patient has not had time to become significantly dehydrated or glycogen depleted. This is called *acute hypothermia*, and spontaneous rewarming is usually possible once the patient has been removed from the water, dried, and insulated.

In slow onset cases, called *sub-acute hypothermia*,

glycogen stores and blood sugar are often depleted. The patient is usually dehydrated. The temperature difference between shell and core is not as dramatic. These patients will not be able to rewarm without help. In fact, rewarming efforts can be lethal without hydration and food.

The most obvious signs of mild hypothermia are mental status changes and shivering. The patient may be lethargic, withdrawn, confused, or exhibit other personality changes. The skin will be pale and cool and there may be some loss of dexterity in the extremities as the shell/core compensation reduces blood flow. Body core temperature will measure below 35° C. Shivering can be mild to severe. If the patient is not already dehydrated, cold diuresis will continue with the patient producing relatively dilute urine.

VITAL SIGNS IN MILD HYPOTHERMIA

P:	Normal to slightly elevated.
BP:	Normal.
R:	Normal.
T:	32 - 35° C.
C:	A to V on AVPU, Mild to moderate MS changes.
S:	Shell/Core compensation.

The most accurate body core temperature measurements are made by esophageal probe, not usually available for field rescue. Rectal measurements would be the next most useful. A special low reading clinical thermometer is required for measuring core temperature below 34° C. Oral, ear, and skin surface measurements are frequently inaccurate in hypothermia.

TREATMENT OF MILD HYPOTHERMIA

Mild hypothermia is an urgent problem requiring immediate and aggressive treatment in the field. The anticipated problem, severe hypothermia, will be much more difficult to handle. The treatment is essentially the same as that for cold response; protect

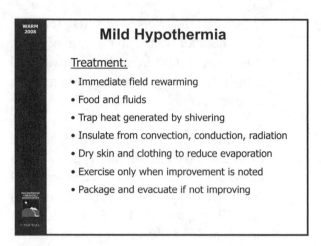

Mild Hypothermia

Treatment:
• Immediate field rewarming
• Food and fluids
• Trap heat generated by shivering
• Insulate from convection, conduction, radiation
• Dry skin and clothing to reduce evaporation
• Exercise only when improvement is noted
• Package and evacuate if not improving

from heat loss and restore calories and fluid.

Vigorous shivering is the most efficient form of field rewarming for the mildly hypothermic patient. It just needs fluid and fuel. Adding external heat with hot water bottles or body heaters is generally safe and certainly more comfortable, but no attempt to mobilize and exercise the patient should be made until obvious improvement in mental status is noted, especially in cases of sub-acute hypothermia.

All hypothermic patients experience some degree of afterdrop, where the body core temperature continues to decrease even after rewarming has begun. This is due to the physics of heat transfer through any medium, but is exacerbated by vasodilatation of the body shell and circulation of blood through the cooler extremities as the patient rewarms. As a result, your patient may get a little worse before getting better, especially if you exercise him too soon which seem to cause a greater degree of afterdrop. It may require over 40 minutes of shivering, sugar, fluids, and aggressive external rewarming before it becomes safe to allow the patient to exercise.

SEVERE HYPOTHERMIA

For hospital treatment, several distinct stages of hypothermia are defined to guide the resuscitation effort. Most commonly these are referred to as mild, moderate, and severe. For field treatment, however, the distinction is mostly practical: can the patient cooperate with your treatment or not? A very cold patient who is not awake and cannot cooperate with

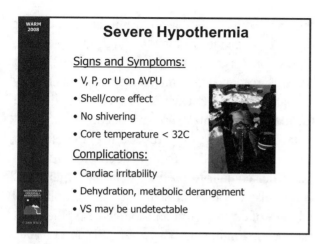

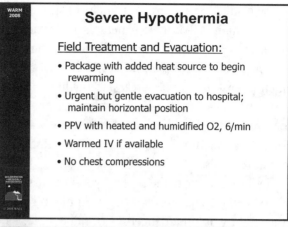

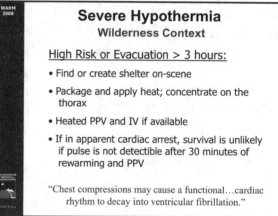

treatment is treated as severely hypothermic. An accurate measurement of core temperature is not required.

As the core temperature falls below 32° C, mental status changes will become severe followed by a drop to V, P, or U on the AVPU scale. This is quite different from the subdued but awake mild hypothermic. Shivering will stop as muscles are deactivated by shell cooling and lack of calories to burn. Cold diureses may continue if fluid stores are not yet depleted.

VITAL SIGNS IN SEVERE HYPOTHERMIA

P:	Slow. May be undetectable.
BP:	Low. May be unobtainable.
R:	Slow. May not be observable.
T:	Below 30–32° C.
C:	Severe MS changes leading to decreased consciousness.
S:	Cold, pale, weak or absent shivering.

TREATMENT OF SEVERE HYPOTHERMIA

The ideal treatment for severe hypothermia is controlled rewarming in a hospital, preferably a level one trauma center. Take the time to properly package the patient before initiating a gentle but urgent evacuation. This should include heat sources such as

warm water bottles or a charcoal heat pack applied to the thorax. This will minimize heat loss and may actually begin rewarming, improving the stability of the cardiovascular system. Rough handling can cause the cold heart to go into ventricular fibrillation. Keep the patient horizontal.

Positive pressure ventilation with heated air may also help. Since the patient's oxygen demand and production of CO_2 is decreased, the rate can be reduced to about six breaths per minute. Intravenous normal saline warmed to 40° C can restore fluid volume without contributing to heat loss.

In extremely cold patients, pulse and respiration may not be detectable. It is quite possible to mistake severe hypothermia for death. Anecdotal experience and animal studies suggests that even patients in apparent cardiopulmonary arrest may be salvageable if the body core temperature is above 10° C and definitive medical care can be accessed within three hours. However, any significant risk to rescuers will not be justified by the low probability of success.

Performing CPR on these patients is of questionable value, may be harmful, and will delay evacuation to definitive care. Chest compressions may cause a functioning but very slow cardiac rhythm to decay into ventricular fibrillation. For these reasons, chest compressions should be performed only where evacuation will not be impeded and a palpable or monitored pulse was suddenly lost.

Field rewarming of the severe hypothermic should be considered as a last resort to be applied if timely evacuation would be dangerous or impossible. Find shelter and apply heat any way that you can, but do not use aggressive external rewarming like immersion in a hot spring or exposure to a hot engine room because this may produce vasodilatation and shock. Add sugar orally if the patient rewarms enough to protect the airway. Dextrose can also be added to an IV. If you succeed, recognize that metabolic derangement may be significant and evacuation to medical care is still the ideal when it can be accomplished.

If your patient is in apparent cardiac arrest and you are more than three hours from definitive care, try to warm her enough to produce detectible vital signs. If no pulse or other life-signs are observed after 30 minutes of external heat and warmed PPV, the effort can be discontinued. Where an AED is available, follow the prompts made by the machine. If no shock is indicated and the patient remains pulseless after 30 minutes of rewarming, she has died.

CASE STUDY: HYPOTHERMIA

Scene: Transatlantic voyage aboard 135-foot sailing school vessel 500 miles east of Newfoundland. The weather has been cold, wet, and windy for the past 24 hours.

S: A 20-year-old student was found huddled at the base of the foremast at dawn. He was last seen at watch change at 23:00 the previous day. He appeared to be unconscious. The watch officer was summoned.

O: The student was responsive to painful stimuli. His foul weather gear was open in front, and he was soaked to the waist. A bruise was noted below his left eye. There was no other obvious injury.

Vital Signs at 05:30 were - BP: 110/70, P: 60, R: 10, C: P on AVPU, T: felt cool, Skin: pale. An empty bottle of Dramamine tablets was found in his jacket pocket. According to his medical screening form, the student had no known allergies, he was not on medication and he had no history of significant medical problems. His last meal would have been a snack at 21:00 the previous day.

A: 1. P on AVPU. Consider low blood sugar, hypothermia, traumatic brain injury, toxins.
　　2. Spine cannot be cleared.

P: 1. hypothermia package, external rewarming
　　2. monitor AVPU and airway
　　3. monitor AVPU and respiration
　　4. sugar orally when airway can be protected
　　5. spine stabilization

CASE STUDY: HYPOTHERMIA (CONTINUED)

Discussion: Wet clothing was removed and the patient was wrapped in a sleeping bag. Hot water bottles were rotated into the package. Although the patient was breathing, ventilations were assisted by mouth to mask. A rectal temperature of 31° C was measured, confirming the suspicion of severe hypothermia.

The patient responded to treatment, improved to V on AVPU, and began to shiver. As soon as he was able to take liquids safely, he was given warm tea and honey. After three hours, he was A on AVPU with normal mental status and a normal core temperature. He was able to explain what happened.

There had been no trauma. He had not been climbing the mast. The bruise below his eye had developed after being struck in the face by a flailing jib sheet two days before. He had taken twice the normal dose of Dramamine to treat his sea sickness and fallen asleep in the location where he had been found.

Although this problem could have been avoided, it was handled appropriately once discovered. The watch officer's plan initially considered all of the possible causes of reduced level of consciousness, including severe hypothermia. As the patient responded to treatment, the other causes could be ruled out by exam and history leaving only the hypothermia and successful recovery.

HEAT RELATED ILLNESS

Because vital organs work best at a temperature of around 37° C, the body will conserve only as much heat as it needs to keep it there and get rid of the rest. Your primary mechanism for heat dissipation is skin vasodilatation and sweat. When sweat evaporates, it absorbs a tremendous amount of heat energy from the skin surface. This is a very effective cooling system as long as there is enough blood and sweat to keep it going. The body constantly sacrifices fluid to maintain normal temperature in hot environments.

Like cold response, heat response is a normal process. As long as heat dissipation can keep up with heat production, the body core temperature will remain normal. Heat response should be treated with fluid replacement and reduction in heat exposure and production. In the backcountry setting, heat response carries the anticipated problems of heat exhaustion and heat stroke.

Sweat can evaporate so quickly in dry climates that profuse sweating may go unnoticed until fluid loss is severe. Pay special attention to fluid replacement when the signs of heat response are present. Reduced urine output is a good indicator that the body is compensating for reduced fluid intake or increased losses. In most circumstances, thirst is also a reliable sign of inadequate fluid intake.

HEAT EXHAUSTION

Heat exhaustion is dehydration from sweating. Body core temperature is normal to slightly elevated. The primary problem is compensated volume shock. The patient will be awake with normal mental status, but often complains of nausea, headache, and weakness. History will reveal inadequate food

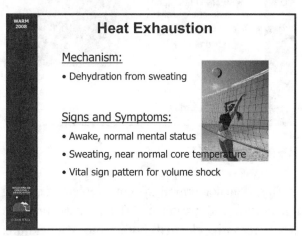

and fluid intake, and reduced urine output. Like any other form of shock, heat exhaustion can be a serious problem that requires immediate treatment in the field.

TREATMENT OF HEAT EXHAUSTION

Stop the fluid loss and replace fluid volume. Move the patient into a cooler area and stop physical exertion to stop sweating. Oral fluid replacement is usually effective, but intravenous fluid is faster. If the patient is vomiting, oral replacement is still possible by giving fluid frequently in small amounts. Look for increased urine production, improved sense of well-being, and normal vital signs as an indication of the return of normal fluid volume. Without IV fluids, it may take more than 12 hours to bring the dehydrated patient back to normal.

The patient may also be salt depleted from sweating. Rehydration with water alone can dilute the remaining salt in the blood causing the problem known as exertional hyponatremia (discussed in more detail later in this chapter). Salt replacement can be accomplished with food or electrolyte drinks. Do not give salt tablets; they will cause stomach irritation and vomiting.

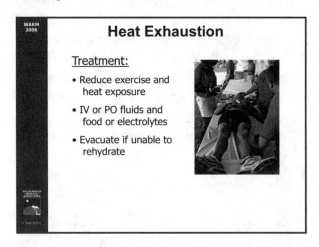

HEAT STROKE

This is major critical system problem requiring immediate field treatment. The primary problem is dangerously elevated body core temperature, which is capable of significant damage to the central nervous system and other vital organs. Radical cooling

is required. The patient may also be in volume shock from dehydration, but this is not the focus of immediate field treatment.

The mechanism of injury may be extreme heat production from vigorous exercise or exposure to high ambient temperatures. Generally it is some combination of the two, like fire fighting or a forced march in hot weather. The patient may have become heat exhausted first, or progressed directly to heat stroke. Medications can also play an important role. People taking diuretics and psychotropic medications are at greater risk of developing heat stroke and other heat-related problems.

Severe mental status changes will rapidly lead to a drop on the AVPU scale. The skin may have the classic hot, red, and dry appearance, but this is not always the case. With extreme heat exposure, a critical rise in core temperature can occur before the patient has time to become dehydrated. The skin may be still wet with sweat. The patient will feel hot.

TREATMENT OF HEAT STROKE

Immediate, radical cooling is required. Immersion in cold water is ideal, but not always available. You can also spray the patient with water and fan her with air, taking advantage of evaporative cooling. Look for an improvement in level of consciousness and mental status to indicate the return to a more normal temperature. The ability to actually measure core temperature may be useful here. Beware that cold water immersion can result in a rapid swing toward

Heat Stroke

Treatment:
- Stop exercise, remove from hot environment
- Immediate and radical cooling
- IV or PO fluids and electrolytes
- Evacuation after cooling is ideal
- Evacuation may be non-emergent if vital signs and mental status return to normal
- Long-term care should include hydration for normal urine output

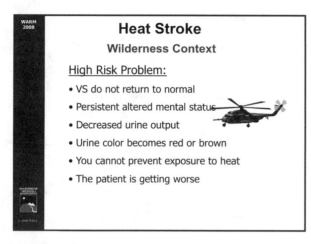

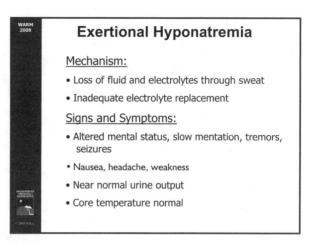

hypothermia.

Fluid replacement is critical, but only after core temperature is being effectively treated. Intravenous fluid replacement is ideal, but oral fluids may work if the patient can cooperate and protect her airway. Advanced life support intervention is a priority.

Emergency evacuation is justified. These patients are best served by treatment and observation in the hospital. Brain injury is possible, with the anticipated problem of elevated ICP. A condition called rhabdomyolysis may develop leading to kidney failure.

Where high-risk evacuation is the only option, transport may be deferred if mental status and other vital signs promptly return to normal. Field care should include rest and aggressive oral hydration to maintain normal urine output. Avoid exertion and heat exposure. Evacuate urgently if urine output decreases or urine becomes red or brown. Also evacuate urgently if the patient begins to feel worse and is unable to take food and fluids or exhibits mental status changes.

EXERTIONAL HYPONATREMIA

Exertional hyponatremia can present as a primary problem in people who have been working or playing hard and drinking large quantities of water. This is a problem most common with extreme athletes and others who are acutely aware of the need to maintain hydration but don't take the time to eat enough. It is magnified in people who are not acclimatized to

the heat and thus are losing excessive amounts of salt through sweat. The patient dilutes the salt content of the body to a point where function is impaired. The term *hyponatremia* means low sodium, one of the body's primary electrolytes.

The signs and symptoms can resemble heat exhaustion with weakness, nausea, and headache, but urine volume is near normal with relatively dilute urine. Hyponatremia typically causes changes in mental status, particularly slow thinking and confusion. But loss of consciousness and seizures can also occur. Tremors are not uncommon.

TREATMENT OF EXERTIONAL HYPONATREMIA

Water restriction and electrolyte replacement is the usual treatment. Sometimes, improvement is immediate with the ingestion of salty foods. If there is evidence that the patient is also dehydrated, volume

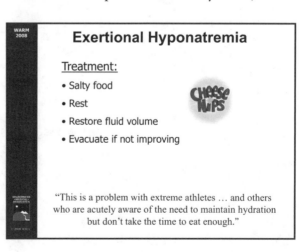

replacement may also be necessary. As with any problem, if the patient is not improving or getting worse, evacuation to medical care is ideal.

NOTES:

Cold Injuries

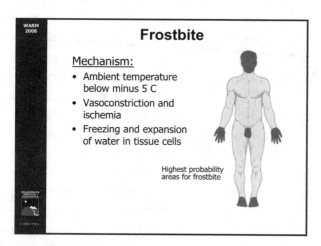

FROSTBITE

The expansion of water as it turns to ice is an impressive natural force. Frost action crumbles mountain ranges, cracks engine blocks, and heaves roads. When freezing occurs in your fingers and toes it is called frostbite, and the effects are no less impressive.

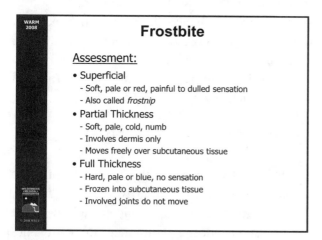

TREATMENT OF SUPERFICIAL FROSTBITE (FROSTNIP)

The superficial stage of frostbite is sometimes called *frostnip*. This occurs with the intense vasoconstriction

and loss of local tissue perfusion that results from exposure to sub-freezing temperatures. The patient may not be aware of the problem, but sensation to touch is usually intact and occasionally painful. The area will appear pink or white, but still feel soft to the touch. You will not yet see ice crystal formation on the surface.

In superficial frostbite, only the outer layers of skin are affected and damage is minimal because ice crystals have not yet formed inside the skin cells. Prompt rewarming at this stage does not result in disability or tissue loss. Simply covering the area and warming the patient to reverse shell/core compensation is usually enough. The patient may experience mild inflammation and pain. There will be no blister formation, but the area may be more susceptible to cold injury for a while.

TREATMENT OF PARTIAL-THICKNESS FROSTBITE

Partial-thickness frostbite occurs when the water in skin cells begins to freeze. Sensation will be dulled, and the area will appear white or blue and feel doughy to the touch. Because subcutaneous tissue is not yet involved, the skin will still move easily over joints and

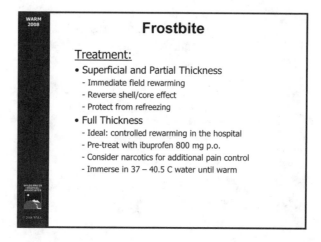

soft tissue. But at this point, the damage has begun. Since water expands in volume as it solidifies, cells and blood vessels suffer mechanical trauma during the freezing process.

Like frostnip, the treatment for partial-thickness frostbite is immediate field rewarming. Cover the area and feed, hydrate, and warm the patient. The rewarmed area will likely be red and sore, and may develop superficial blisters. Continued care includes wound management and protection from refreezing. Long-term disability is unlikely, but scar formation in the injured tissue can cause an increased lifelong susceptibility to frostbite.

TREATMENT OF FULL-THICKNESS FROSTBITE

Full-thickness frostbite is a serious injury. The skin and underlying tissues are frozen solid. The area is white or bluish and firm to touch. The skin does not move over joints or underlying tissues. Ice crystals are usually visible on the skin surface and there is a complete loss of sensation. The digit or extremity feels like a club.

Full-thickness frostbite is best rewarmed under controlled conditions in a medical facility. Much of the tissue damage from prolonged or very deep freezing occurs during and after rewarming. Inflammation, pain and infection are anticipated problems. Rewarmed tissue is very susceptible to further injury, even from normal use. Refreezing is devastating. Allowing tissue to remain frozen for several hours

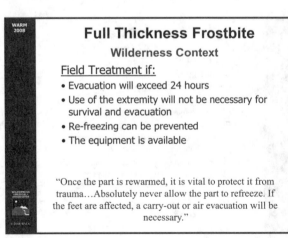

Full Thickness Frostbite

Wilderness Context

Field Treatment if:

- Evacuation will exceed 24 hours
- Use of the extremity will not be necessary for survival and evacuation
- Re-freezing can be prevented
- The equipment is available

"Once the part is rewarmed, it is vital to protect it from trauma…Absolutely never allow the part to refreeze. If the feet are affected, a carry-out or air evacuation will be necessary."

during a self-evacuation is better than walking out on rewarmed feet.

If you find yourself stuck somewhere that makes evacuation impossible within about twenty four hours, field rewarming may be your only option. Set up a secure shelter and be sure your patient is warm, dry, well fed, and hydrated. Pre-medicate with an anti-inflammatory drug like ibuprofen (800 milligrams) taken by mouth. This will reduce pain and inflammation and help prevent blood clots in the rewarmed tissue. Giving stronger pain medication may be necessary during the process.

Spontaneous rewarming can be accelerated by immersing the frozen extremity in water warmed to $37 - 40\,^{\circ}$ C. The water should feel hot to normal skin, but not uncomfortable. Keep adding warm water to the pot to keep the temperature up as the thawing process continues. Avoid direct exposure to dry heat like a camp fire.

Once the part is rewarmed, it is vital to protect it from trauma. This means no use of the digit or extremity. Absolutely never allow the part to refreeze. If the feet are affected, a carry-out or air evacuation will be necessary. Rewarmed frostbite is a high-risk wound. Early surgical referral is indicated.

Monitor distal CSM frequently to ensure that splints or bandages do not constrict circulation as swelling develops. If possible, keep the part elevated. Continue regular doses of ibuprofen. If you have it, cover the area with aloe vera gel or ointment, which has been shown to have both anti-inflammatory and anti-bacterial properties.

PREVENTION OF FROSTBITE

Anything which restricts the circulation of warm blood to tissues allows freezing to occur more readily. In people who are already a little chilled, shell/core compensation reduces perfusion to the extremities to maintain core temperature. Constricting clothing such as ski boots or a splint tied too tightly can reduce blood flow as well. Cigarette smoking is additional factor, infusing the body tissues with nicotine, which is a powerful vasoconstrictor.

Certainly, well-insulated and fitted boots, gloves, and a face mask can go a long way toward preventing frostbite in extreme conditions. But equally important is maintaining an active and warm body core. This will ensure a good supply of warm blood to the extremities. That's why you eat a good breakfast and wear a hat to keep your feet warm.

TRENCH FOOT

Trench foot is an injury that develops with prolonged exposure to cold and wet conditions above freezing. It is not limited to feet and often involves the hands of paddlers, fisherman, and others working or playing on the water. Inflammation is a results from prolonged vasoconstriction and tissue breakdown, an example of ischemia to infarction. Blisters can develop, with the possibility of secondary infection where the dermis has been exposed.

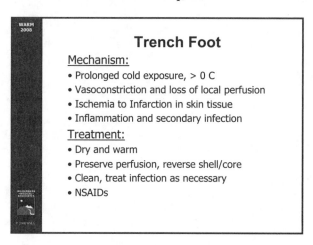

Trench Foot

Mechanism:
- Prolonged cold exposure, > 0 C
- Vasoconstriction and loss of local perfusion
- Ischemia to Infarction in skin tissue
- Inflammation and secondary infection

Treatment:
- Dry and warm
- Preserve perfusion, reverse shell/core
- Clean, treat infection as necessary
- NSAIDs

TREATMENT OF TRENCH FOOT (OR HAND)

Since the mechanism is ischemia from being wet and cold, the basic treatment is to increase perfusion by keeping the feet warm and dry. Treat any open wounds to prevent infection and allow for healing. Ibuprofen may help with inflammation and pain. Like rewarmed frostbite, tissue damage can be exacerbated by further use. Walking may become difficult or impossible.

Prevention is worth the trouble. In "trench" conditions, try to give your hands and feet several dry and warm hours each day. Reverse shell/core compensation by maintaining hydration, calories, and activity. It's okay to dry your wet socks in your sleeping bag at night, but not while wearing them. Take your wetsuit booties and gloves off whenever possible. Inside waterproof boots, change your socks frequently to keep your feet as dry as you can.

RAYNAUD'S PHENOMENON

Raynaud's is a disorder of the blood vessels in the hands and fingers aggravated by cold exposure. Profound vasoconstriction causes temporary ischemia, with the typical white or blue appearance and numbness and tingling. It is usually self-limiting if the extremity is protected from further cold exposure. Pre-disposing factors include repetitive use injury, vibration injury, and previous cold injury. Raynaud's can also be a feature of other systemic illness.

Our primary concern in backcountry medicine is that Raynaud's patients are at high risk for frostbite in freezing weather and for prolonged ischemia in cool weather, with the attendant tissue breakdown and inflammation. These people need to be especially conscientious about wearing gloves and staying warm and well hydrated. Definitive treatment is prolonged and may involve the use of medication and desensitizing exposure to cold and hot stimulus.

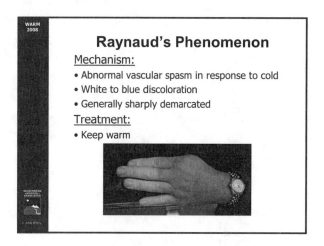

Raynaud's Phenomenon

Mechanism:
- Abnormal vascular spasm in response to cold
- White to blue discoloration
- Generally sharply demarcated

Treatment:
- Keep warm

NOTES:

Altitude Illness

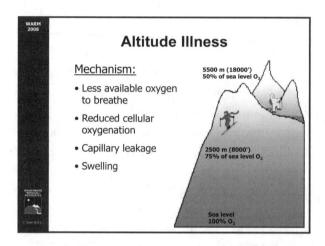

Altitude Illness

Mechanism:

- Less available oxygen to breathe
- Reduced cellular oxygenation
- Capillary leakage
- Swelling

5500 m (18000')
50% of sea level O_2

2500 m (8000')
75% of sea level O_2

Sea level
100% O_2

As you climb in elevation, the atmosphere becomes less dense and, as a result, provides less oxygen for each breath. It is this decrease in available oxygen that causes the most important altitude-related symptoms. At sea level, a healthy respiratory system will nearly completely fill the hemoglobin in the red blood cells with oxygen, yielding an oxygen saturation measurement of 98–100%. As altitude increases, oxygen saturation begins to decrease. At an altitude of 3000 meters, oxygen saturation typically measures 90–96%. For most people from sea level, this represents mild hypoxia that can result in a noticeable decrease in performance and at least minimal symptoms of altitude illness.

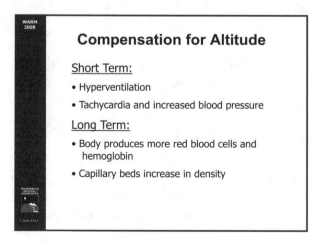

Compensation for Altitude

Short Term:

- Hyperventilation
- Tachycardia and increased blood pressure

Long Term:

- Body produces more red blood cells and hemoglobin
- Capillary beds increase in density

Initially, the body compensates with mild hyperventilation and increased cardiac output. This is observed as an increased respiratory rate, increased pulse rate, and mildly elevated blood pressure. This allows for a person to ascend, within limits, without a significant reduction in cellular oxygenation.

One side effect of the body's compensatory effort is respiratory alkalosis, a rise in blood pH due to increased respiration. This produces some of the commonly felt altitude symptoms such as sleep

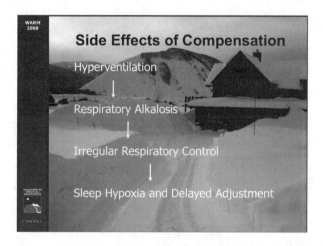

Side Effects of Compensation

Hyperventilation
↓
Respiratory Alkalosis
↓
Irregular Respiratory Control
↓
Sleep Hypoxia and Delayed Adjustment

hypoxia. The increased respiratory rate allows more carbon dioxide to escape the blood plasma into the expired air. Carbon dioxide is a waste product of cellular metabolism and is transported as a dissolved gas in the blood plasma. Getting rid of more of it might seem beneficial, but carbon dioxide also has an important role in maintaining the acid/base balance in the blood, normally kept at a pH of 7.43.

Under normal conditions, your brain monitors changes in pH as the primary method of controlling respiratory effort. The brain should respond to a rise in pH by reducing the rate and depth of respiration to retain more carbon dioxide. But at altitude, this response is in conflict with the need to extract more oxygen from thinner air. The result is often a disturbance in the breathing pattern, particularly during sleep when breathing normally slows. It also inhibits the adjustment process.

As part of the short-term adjustment, the kidneys excrete bicarbonate (a base) in an attempt to reset the pH balance to the new respiratory rate. This usually takes two or three days, and may or may not be completely successful. Patients can help the process by avoiding higher elevations until adjusted, and maintaining adequate hydration for kidney function. A medication called acetazolamide can help with this process.

Long-term compensation for an individual staying at altitude includes producing more red blood cells to carry oxygen and the development of more dense capillary beds in body tissues. This process can take months to years. The acclimatized individual's oxygen saturation will still read low, but because the carrying capacity of the blood has increased, there is actually more oxygen being transported.

Alpinists can continue to ascend as long as they allow enough time for short- and long-term adjustment. How quickly this occurs and how high a person can ultimately go depend on health, fitness, and genetics. Eventually, the ability to compensate is maximized and inadequate cellular oxygenation will prevent further ascent.

ALTITUDE ILLNESS

Reduced oxygen in the blood and body tissues results in edema due to capillary dilation and leakage. This generally occurs as oxygen saturation falls below about 90%. The mechanism is not completely understood and is different in the brain than in the lungs. But, the signs and symptoms we worry most about are the same as those seen in cerebral or pulmonary edema from other causes.

High Altitude Cerebral Edema (HACE) is caused by vascular dilation and increased blood flow that result in capillary leakage of fluid into the brain. High Altitude Pulmonary Edema (HAPE) is the result of pulmonary artery constriction causing pulmonary

hypertension. This has the effect of forcing fluid to leak from capillary beds in the lungs into the alveoli.

HACE looks similar to elevated ICP from a TBI or any other cause of brain tissue damage. The signs and symptoms of HAPE are similar to those of pulmonary edema from heart problems, infection, or drowning events.

HACE

The symptoms of mild HACE are often called acute mountain sickness. A small amount of cerebral edema produces the characteristic headache, loss of appetite, and nausea associated with the slight increase in ICP. These are the same symptoms one might expect following a mild TBI. Acute mountain sickness generally develops within a few hours of arrival at moderate altitudes and resolves within 48 hours for most people.

Treatment is largely symptomatic. Aspirin, ibuprofen, or another aspirin-like drug will reduce

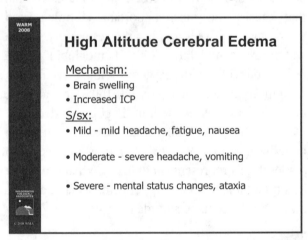

High Altitude Cerebral Edema

Mechanism:
• Brain swelling
• Increased ICP

S/sx:
• Mild - mild headache, fatigue, nausea

• Moderate - severe headache, vomiting

• Severe - mental status changes, ataxia

pain, and may actually reduce cerebral edema. Hydration will be important to kidney function, and the patient should avoid alcohol and narcotic medication that would depress respiratory drive. The prescription drug acetazolamide can be used to reduce symptoms by maintaining a more normal blood pH.

Ideally, a climber should not continue to ascend until symptoms have resolved. However, schedules often interfere with ideal prevention and treatment.

Pushing through symptoms to a higher altitude or level of activity can make the situation much worse.

Moderate HACE is caused by increased intracranial pressure due to brain swelling. The patient will show early mental status changes and begin to vomit. The headache may not respond to NSAIDs. The ideal treatment is supplemental oxygen, and an immediate descent of at least 300 meters.

If the patient is pinned down by weather or terrain, treatment in place includes rest, pain medication, supplemental oxygen, and fluid to maintain hydration. For a short time under emergency circumstances a steroidal anti-inflammatory can be used to reduce the symptoms of cerebral edema. An example is the drug dexamethasone, given by mouth or intramuscular injection.

A portable hyperbaric chamber (e.g., Gamow Bag) is another emergency treatment occasionally available through rescue teams or cached at popular climbing areas. This device can be used to temporarily increase the air pressure around the patient by about two pounds per square inch, simulating a decent of 1000–2000 meters. This may temporarily improve the patient's condition allowing a walk-out evacuation before debilitating symptoms reoccur.

The symptoms of moderate HACE may improve with treatment and time. But, climbing partners or rescuers must be prepared for an emergency descent if the patient's condition worsens. The practitioner must also be alert to other anticipated problems such as hypothermia and volume shock from dehydration.

Severe HACE is a major critical system problem.

Fortunately, it rarely occurs below 4000 meters in elevation. One of the common signs is ataxia (unable to walk straight). The patient will also exhibit changes in level of consciousness and mental status that may range from mild to profound. Persistent vomiting and complete loss of appetite are common.

The symptoms of severe HACE can be confused with those of other problems such as hypoglycemia, dehydration, hypothermia, hyperthermia, and simple exhaustion. All of these problems can cause a decrease in muscular performance and efficiency and all can cause changes in mental status. Even though your primary concern may be altitude, it is important to include all five problems as possible causes until proven otherwise.

Severe HACE is treated using all the techniques and medications useful for the mild and moderate forms, plus an immediate descent of at least 1000 meters. Exertion should be minimized, but there should be no delay in descent. A patient in severe HACE is not likely to survive without aggressive intervention.

HIGH ALTITUDE PULMONARY EDEMA (HAPE)

Unlike HACE that develops within 24 hours, HAPE tends to develop several days after arrival at altitude. It can exist without any symptoms of HACE, or present long after symptoms of HACE have cleared. At moderate altitudes (3000–4000 meters), HAPE tends to occur as an isolated illness.

The initial symptoms of HAPE are shortness

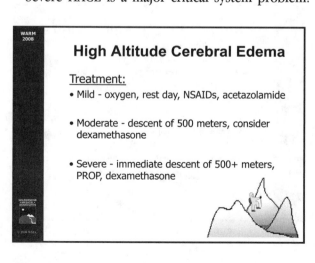

High Altitude Cerebral Edema

Treatment:
- Mild - oxygen, rest day, NSAIDs, acetazolamide

- Moderate - descent of 500 meters, consider dexamethasone

- Severe - immediate descent of 500+ meters, PROP, dexamethasone

High Altitude Pulmonary Edema

Mechanism:
- Swelling of lung tissue
- Leakage of fluid into the alveoli

S/sx:
- Mild HAPE - dry cough, mild SOB on exertion
- Moderate HAPE - persistent cough, crackles on auscultation, SOB at rest, low grade fever
- Severe HAPE – mental status changes, respiratory failure, blood-tinged sputum, marked crackles

of breath on exertion and a dry cough. It can also produce a low-grade fever. People with an existing or recent respiratory illness seem to be more predisposed to develop HAPE. In fact, many patients will mistake mild HAPE for a worsening pneumonia or bronchitis. In the early stages, fluid in the alveoli may not be audible with a stethoscope.

The ideal treatment for HAPE is supplemental oxygen and immediate descent. Significant improvement or resolution of symptoms can be noted with as little as 300 meters drop in altitude. Mild HAPE can also be safely managed on-site if low-flow supplemental oxygen can be given over 24 hours, and descent will be easy and quick to accomplish if conditions worsen. Acetazolamide at 125 mg twice a day may also help.

As pulmonary edema worsens, the patient will experience shortness of breath even at rest and a persistent cough. Crackles will be audible with a

High Altitude Pulmonary Edema

Treatment:
- Mild HAPE - oxygen, rest day, hydration and food, acetazolamide

- Moderate HAPE - immediate descent of 500 meters, consider nifedipine

- Severe HAPE - PROP, immediate descent of 500+ meters, nifedipine or tadalafil

stethoscope or an ear to the chest. Moderate HAPE is a bad sign. The condition tends to progress from bad to worse.

Unfortunately, exertion will make pulmonary edema worse due to an increase in pulmonary hypertension. There may be situations where it would be better to remain where you are rather than perform a strenuous evacuation over a mountain pass. If decent will be delayed, supplemental oxygen and positive pressure ventilations can be lifesaving. HAPE will also respond to treatment in a portable hyperbaric chamber.

Emergency medications for HAPE include oral nifedipine, a smooth muscle relaxer that is normally used to treat high blood pressure. It seems to ease the pulmonary hypertension that is forcing fluid to leak into the alveolar space. Nifedipine is a prescription medication in the United States. There is also emerging evidence that inhaled albuterol can prevent or treat HAPE, although this treatment is not yet in common use.

Severe HAPE will ultimately result in respiratory failure and death. Emergency treatment includes PPV, oxygen, nifedipine, and an immediate descent of at least 1000 meters. Pulmonary edema may persist for several days after descent and require hospital observation and treatment. Unlike HACE, severe HAPE is seen at moderate altitudes between 2800 and 4000 meters.

OTHER ALTITUDE ILLNESS

While HACE and HAPE are the most dangerous forms of altitude illness; they are not the only manifestation. Capillary dilation and leakage can produce edema anywhere in the body. People traveling at altitude can end up with edematous hand and feet. Swelling in the gut can produce diarrhea. Edema in the mucous membranes of the nose and sinuses can mimic the congestion of a cold or sinus infection. Altitude will make the symptoms of an existing illness worse. The reduction in available oxygen as well as the reduced protective effects of the atmosphere predisposes people to other problems as well.

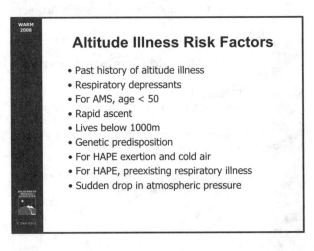

Altitude Illness Risk Factors

- Past history of altitude illness
- Respiratory depressants
- For AMS, age < 50
- Rapid ascent
- Lives below 1000m
- Genetic predisposition
- For HAPE exertion and cold air
- For HAPE, preexisting respiratory illness
- Sudden drop in atmospheric pressure

Medical Aspects of Avalanche Rescue

19

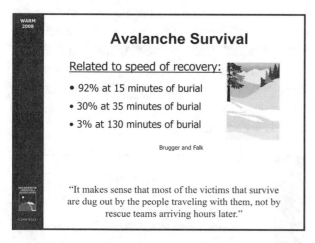

Avalanche Survival

Related to speed of recovery:

• 92% at 15 minutes of burial

• 30% at 35 minutes of burial

• 3% at 130 minutes of burial

Brugger and Falk

"It makes sense that most of the victims that survive are dug out by the people traveling with them, not by rescue teams arriving hours later."

Of avalanche fatalities, 15% are caused by trauma and about 5% by hypothermia. The rest die of asphyxia. The most important factor in survival of avalanche burial is the speed of recovery. Statistics vary, but in the first fifteen minutes between 80 and 90% of victims are found alive. This drops to about 30% at 35 minutes and around 3% at 130 minutes. It makes sense that most of the victims that survive are dug out by the people traveling with them, not by rescue teams arriving hours later.

RECOVERY

Survival of prolonged burial is rare, but documented. These are the cases where the victim comes to rest in an air space around a tree or boulder, or has been partially protected by building debris. Also, new backcountry safety equipment such as the Avalung can allow victims to continue breathing under the snow for an hour or more. The possibility of a prolonged survival, however slim, makes avalanche search and recovery a high-priority mission.

Again, statistics vary from place to place, but all data indicate that survival is highly unlikely when burial is deeper than two meters. That's why most avalanche probes carried by backcountry skiers are less than three meters long. The longer and heavier probes are carried only by rescue teams performing body recovery.

The most efficient tool for locating a buried victim is a well-trained avalanche search dog team but these rarely arrive on-scene soon enough to make a difference. If the victim is wearing an avalanche beacon, other members of the group may be able to find and recover him within minutes. If neither dog nor beacon is available, a live-find is unlikely unless some part of the victim is projecting above the surface of the snow. The backup plan consists of a probe line of rescuers working slowly through the debris field.

There are a number of other devices being tested and used in avalanche recovery. Metal detectors are useful for locating snow machines or skis, which may or may not be near the buried victim. The Recco System used in some ski areas is a device that broadcasts a directional radio wave that excites a small metallic tag or sticker sewn into the skiers clothing. The "reflected" signal is picked up by the unit's receiver and can be followed directly back to the victim. The device has been known to detect a reflected signal off of cell phones, radios, and other metallic objects.

If a live victim is recovered, the primary problem addressed by the medical officer will be respiratory arrest due to asphyxiation. This can occur as a result of snow packed into the nose and mouth, the formation of an ice mask, or restricted respiratory excursion due to the pressure of the snow pack.

Snow is mostly air and is very porous. Unless the airway is packed with snow, the victim may be able to breathe for a period of time. Eventually, the victim's exhaled breath will condense and freeze into a nonporous ice mask around the airway. This effect may be delayed by the use of an Avalung or the good fortune to have large air space formed by vegetation or debris. For these reasons, an avalanche recovery is still considered an urgent response even if it will take a rescue team an hour or more to reach the scene.

TREATMENT

The treatment includes immediate PPV, supplemental oxygen, and evacuation. Once the patient is freed from the snow pack, hypothermia becomes an anticipated problem. Airway control is critical if the patient is less than A on AVPU. Increased ICP due to brain hypoxia can also develop, but this is likely to occur well after an evacuation has been accomplished.

The resuscitation of an avalanche victim in full cardiopulmonary arrest should not be attempted if there is obvious lethal injury or the effort puts rescuers at risk. Experience shows that the chances of success are minimal after 30 minutes of complete burial. If the victim's airway is packed with snow, you can assume that breathing stopped at the time the avalanche occurred.

Drawing the line between treating a patient and performing a body recovery can be a difficult decision to make. If you choose to begin CPR, the effort may be discontinued after 30 minutes of pulselessness. If the equipment is available, a cardiac monitor showing asystole or an AED that refuses to shock a pulseless patient would also confirm that the patient has died.

Hypothermia is not an immediate problem or benefit to the completely buried victim. Respiratory failure will kill the victim long before any protective effect of severe hypothermia is realized. There is no reason to extend the resuscitation beyond the 30-minute CPR protocol or to evacuate and rewarm a pulseless victim as a severe hypothermic. The only exception might be a recovery after many hours or days from a buried building or vehicle with a large preserved air space.

Avalanche awareness and search and recovery are major topics in their own right. Practitioners working with SAR teams in avalanche terrain must be trained and equipped for safe travel and operation. Avalanche recovery represents a considerable risk to rescuers, often in cases where the chance for a live find is minimal. Unfortunately, training in avalanche awareness alone is not enough to prevent an accident. Many people who end up buried are well aware of avalanche risks. In the end, sound judgment on-scene is everything.

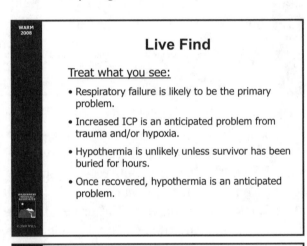

Submersion Injury

Drowning is death by asphyxiation due to submersion, usually in water. Your ability to swim has little to do with your ability to drown. One common cause of drowning is the loss of muscular coordination due to the rapid shell cooling that occurs in cold water. Sometimes, sudden immersion in very cold water causes a reflex gasp that fills the lungs and immediately deprives the victim of oxygen. Swimming and extrication efforts may be hampered by bulky clothing and boots or by being pinned down by a fast current. Even the strongest swimmer can drown in these conditions. Most of the time, a substantial amount of water enters the lungs. In about 15% of cases, the larynx goes into spasm, closing off the lungs and resulting in a *dry drowning*.

The term submersion injury implies survival, at least temporarily. Most people who survive submersion and water inhalation rescue themselves. An event with self rescue, no loss of consciousness, and no persistent respiratory symptoms is not likely to result in critical system problems. This patient may be uncomfortable and scared, but is not in trouble. It is the patient who has lost consciousness and had to be rescued and resuscitated that you should worry most about.

TREATMENT OF SUBMERSION INJURY

The initial assessment problem is respiratory arrest, and the immediate treatment is positive pressure ventilation. There is no need to drain water from the lungs, and there is no difference in field treatment between salt and fresh water. If the effort is initiated within a few minutes of submersion, the patient may recover spontaneous respiration quickly.

You can now congratulate yourself for the save, but should begin an urgent evacuation with the anticipated problem of respiratory failure from pulmonary edema and elevated ICP from cerebral edema. Water inhalation causes irritation of the alveoli in the lungs. Hypoxia causes brain injury. In all but the warmest water, hypothermia can also become an issue.

People who are submerged for more than a few minutes will go into cardiac arrest. At that point, successful field resuscitation is highly unlikely. The few survivors of prolonged submersion have benefited from the effects of very cold water where rapid cooling of the brain delays the damage caused by hypoxia. In rare cases, patients have been resuscitated after

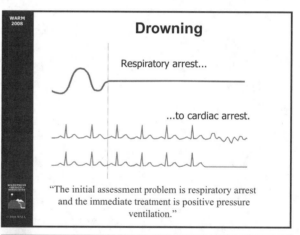

"The initial assessment problem is respiratory arrest and the immediate treatment is positive pressure ventilation."

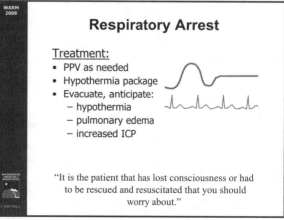

"It is the patient that has lost consciousness or had to be rescued and resuscitated that you should worry about."

an hour of submersion. The best chance for survival occurs with young patients submerged in near-freezing fresh water in close proximity to sophisticated medical care.

In the remote setting, an attempt at resuscitation following prolonged submersion of up to an hour should only be made if it does not place rescuers at risk. Patients who do not respond quickly to basic life support do not survive. Resuscitation efforts beyond the 30-minute CPR or AED protocols are not justified.

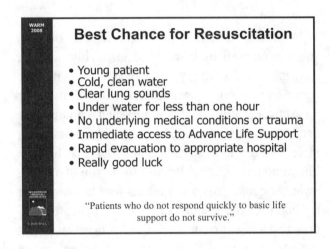

NOTES:

SCUBA Diving Injuries

21

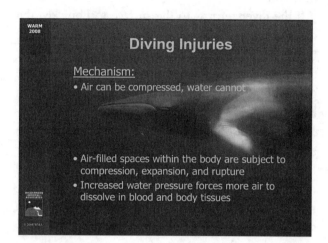

Diving Injuries

Mechanism:
- Air can be compressed, water cannot

- Air-filled spaces within the body are subject to compression, expansion, and rupture
- Increased water pressure forces more air to dissolve in blood and body tissues

Diving Principles

BOYLE'S LAW: $P = 1/v$

HENRY'S LAW: $\uparrow P = \uparrow$ Volume Gas in Solution

	Boyle's Law	Henry's Law
depth/pressure	gas volume	dissolved gas
1 atm. (sea level)	normal	normal
2 atm. (10m)	1/2 normal	2 x normal
3 atm. (20m)	1/3 normal	3 x normal
4 atm. (30m)	1/4 normal	4 x normal

Hyperbaric injury was largely unknown before the invention of Self Contained Underwater Breathing Apparatus (SCUBA). Only a few cases were seen from diving bells and in workers from pressurized bridge construction caissons until the emergence of military and sport diving in the 1940s. It took a number of years and a lot of death and disability before the problems associated with breathing gas under pressure were identified and understood.

Certified sport and commercial divers are now well trained in the prevention and recognition of hyperbaric injury. But, because SCUBA has become popular as a tool for both recreation and rescue, it is important for all medical personnel working in water rescue and marine environments to be able to recognize and treat diving injuries. This chapter will serve as an overview for practitioners who have not had the benefit of SCUBA training.

ARTERIAL GAS EMBOLUS AND DECOMPRESSION SICKNESS

Dive-related injuries are caused by the behavior of air under pressure. As described by Boyle's Law, an air-filled balloon forced underwater would be compressed to one half of its original volume at ten meters below the surface. At twenty meters underwater, the balloon will be reduced to a third of its original volume. The same amount of air molecules will still be present, but they will occupy less space. If the balloon is allowed to return to the surface it will expand back to its normal size without damage. This is exactly what happens to the lungs of a free-diver not using pressurized air.

In order to breathe underwater, a diver must be able to expand his lungs against the massive force of water pressure. Doing this more than a half of a meter below the surface requires the assistance of pressurized air. The SCUBA tank and regulator provides just enough air pressure to overcome water pressure and allow the diver to expand his lungs to full volume. At ten meters below the surface, the diver's lungs will contain twice as many air molecules as they would on the surface. The diver could also use his SCUBA tank to pressurize our example balloon to its original volume, even though it is also ten meters underwater.

As the diver swims back toward the surface, our balloon begins to expand as the water pressure lessens. The diver's lungs also begin to expand, but because he continues to breathe as he ascends, the excess volume is vented through the regulator. Since

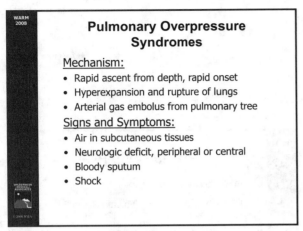

the balloon has no ability to vent, it continues to expand until it ruptures in a cloud of bubbles. This is also what would happen to the lungs of the SCUBA diver if he ascended too fast for the expanding air to escape.

Arterial Gas Embolus (AGE) is the most dramatic and serious of hyperbaric injury. The usual cause is a panic rush for the surface while forgetting to breathe. Expanding air ruptures the lungs and airways, allowing air to enter the subcutaneous tissue and circulatory system. Large bubbles of air can block blood flow, causing ischemia in the heart, brain, and other vital organs. Death can be immediate. If the diver survives, there will be major critical system injury.

The other major diving injury is decompression sickness, otherwise known as *the bends*. This is caused by the tendency of air under pressure to dissolve into the blood and body tissues with which it is in contact. As stated by Henry's Law, the greater the pressure the more air will be dissolved.

As a diver descends, the air she is breathing is forced to dissolve into her blood and tissues in direct proportion to water depth. The deeper she goes and the longer she stays, the more air forced into solution. That's why deeper dives are usually kept shorter in duration.

If the diver returns to the surface too quickly, the gas will come out of solution to form bubbles in the blood. The best illustration of this is the head that forms on your beer when you open the bottle. The gas bubbles out when you release the pressure. In beer, this is good. In the blood, this is bad.

As long as the diver ascends slowly enough, the emerging gas molecules will be expired through her lungs without causing injury. Dive computers and decompression tables are used to determine a safe rate of ascent. This reduces the risk of decompression sickness, but does not eliminate it completely. Off-gassing actually continues for many hours after a dive.

If a diver fails to decompress adequately for the depth and duration of the dive, small bubbles will block blood flow in the smaller vessels. The early symptoms of decompression sickness, such as skin itching, are cause by ischemia at the capillary level. Larger bubbles tend to lodge at joints causing joint pain. Bubbles causing ischemia in the brain can cause the symptoms of stroke. Bubbles in the spinal cord can cause paralysis. The onset of these various symptoms can be delayed by many hours, and will be exacerbated by travel to high altitude or the low cabin pressure in an aircraft.

TREATMENT OF AGE AND DECOMPRESSION SICKNESS

Basic and advanced life support, including the administration of high-flow oxygen, during rapid evacuation to a hyperbaric chamber is the ideal treatment for both AGE and decompression sickness. The Diver's Alert Network (available by phone: 919-684-8111) can help you find one. The chamber is the safest place to pressurize the patient to shrink the bubbles that are causing the problems.

MIDDLE EAR BAROTRAUMA AND MASK SQUEEZE

Middle ear barotraumas is not limited to SCUBA divers; free divers can suffer also. The tympanic membrane in the ear is particularly susceptible to injury from changes in water or air pressure. As the diver descends, he must force air into the middle ear behind the ear drum to counter the water pressure pushing in from the outside. As long as the air pressure inside matches the water pressure outside, the ear drum will remain uninjured. If either becomes excessive, the membrane will rupture and allow water to enter the middle ear.

This is usually not an emergency, but carries the anticipated problem of middle ear infection (discussed in chapter 32). The patient should not be permitted to swim or dive until the ear drum has healed. This usually takes several weeks to months. Serious problems can develop when the injury involves the inner ear or facial nerves. Treatment for these red flag symptoms includes early evacuation to medical care.

Mask squeeze develops from a failure to pressurize the air space in the face mask during descent. The relative increase in pressure in the vascular system and soft tissue under the mask can cause the rupture of small blood vessels in the conjunctiva of the eye and skin of the face and nose. Although scary looking, it is usually not serious. Treatment is directed at relieving symptoms.

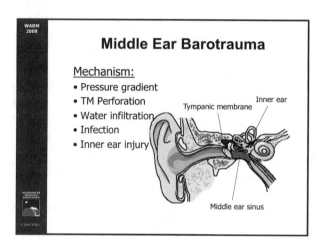

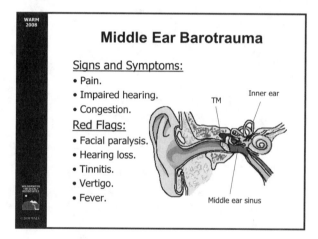

NOTES:

NOTES:

Lightning Injuries

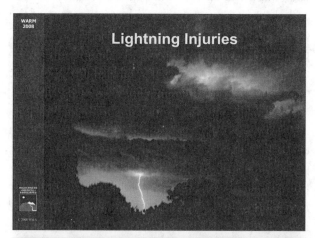

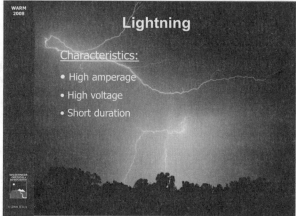

the lower regions of a thunderstorm become more negatively charged, the earth's surface below will become more positively charged. The tendency of similarly-charged objects to repel each other explains why your hair stands on end when you're about to be struck by lightning. Other signs of accumulating electrostatic charge include small rocks jumping about, glowing air around metal objects, and the smell of ozone.

A lightning strike occurs when these charges build up enough potential difference to overcome atmospheric resistance. A conductive column of ionized air is created by stepwise progressions of leader strokes, usually from a negatively charged region, that ultimately meet shorter streamers from the opposite side. The connection allows an electrical discharge generating millions of volts and tens of thousands of amperes. Fortunately, about 95% of lightning passes from cloud to cloud. Only about 5% of lightning activity involves ground strikes.

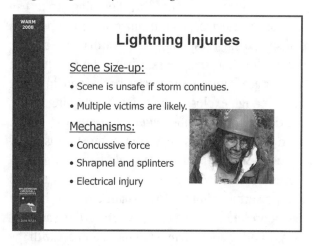

Lightning is nature's way of equalizing the difference in electrostatic charge that develops between regions of the atmosphere and between the atmosphere and the earth's surface during violent weather. Convection caused by ground heating, the advance of a cold front, or air passing over hills and mountains tends to cause an accumulation of positive ions in the cloud tops, negatively charged electrons in the mid cloud, and a weak layer of positive charges in the cloud base. The more violent the convection is, the more rapidly the charges will develop and the more frequent the lightning.

Cumulus clouds showing progressive vertical development indicate the potential for lightning. As

INJURIES

In spite of its massive power, lightning is extremely brief in duration. The average discharge lasts for only about 0.001 seconds. This is not enough time for much

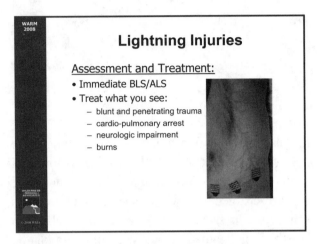

of the electrical energy to overcome skin resistance and enter the body. Less than 20% of lightning victims die of their injuries. Most of the current passes over the skin surface on its way to the ground. As a result, the types of internal injuries typical of manmade electrical current are rarely seen with lightning.

The energy in lightning is dissipated in the form of heat and light. The instantaneous heating and expansion of the column of air through which the current passes generates the shock wave we hear as thunder. Like any explosion, if you are close enough the shock wave can rupture ear drums and fracture bones and damage internal organs. You can also be injured by flying rock, splinters, and other debris.

The direct current flow in a lightning strike can disrupt the electrochemical function of the nervous system, causing respiratory and cardiac arrest. The current flowing over the skin heats the moisture on the surface causing superficial burns and in some cases enough explosive force to blow clothing apart.

A direct hit where the patient becomes part of the main path to ground is likely to be the most devastating. A person can also be injured by splash-over or ground current. Splash-over can be best described as a much less powerful splinter of the main airborne bolt. It may represent involvement in an upward streamer as the ground charge attempts to make contact with the airborne leader stroke.

Ground current spreads out through the earth, rock, or water from "ground zero." It can follow underground roots, pipes, wires, and water courses. Because the energy is diffused, both forms of indirect exposure are generally less devastating than a direct hit.

The extent of injury from current is related to the path the current takes over and through the body. If you're holding onto a steel shroud when the bolt hits your mast, the current may pass through your arm and chest and out your feet. The vital organs of the critical body systems can become part of the path, producing major critical system problems. Ground current usually passes onto one foot and off the other, leaving the vital organs outside the path.

In responding to a lightning injury, the scene size-up for dangers is particularly important. If the storm continues, it may be very dangerous to approach the scene on a hilltop or cliff face. Look for more than one patient; about 9% of lightning injuries involve two or more people. Although it is rare, the explosive force in a direct strike or near miss can cause significant blunt trauma, including ruptured organs and broken bones. Burns caused by lightning are generally superficial, with more serious deep burns occurring in less than 5% of patients. Nervous system disruption is common, with many patients experiencing loss of consciousness, amnesia, and parasthesias. The fatal event is cardiac arrest.

TREATMENT OF LIGHTNING INJURY

Treat what you see. Lightning can induce cardiac arrest. If heart damage is minimal, the pulse will often return spontaneously. Lightning induced respiratory arrest may not spontaneously resolve, even when the respiratory system is relatively intact. In these cases, the prompt initiation of CPR or PPV can be lifesaving. Burns, shock, brain injury, and musculoskeletal trauma are all treated as you would with any other patient. About 25% of survivors will develop significant long-term physical or psychological problems.

PREVENTION OF LIGHTNING INJURY

The height and isolation of an object are the only two factors that predict the likelihood of a lightning strike. The type of material has no influence of the

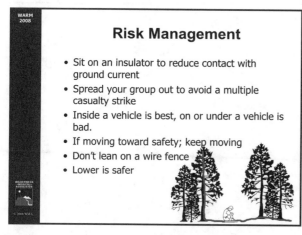

probability of being struck. Metal, however, will do a much better job of conducting the current to ground than wood or plastic. Trees offer higher resistance to the flow of current and will become hot, burn, and may explode as the moisture in the wood instantly vaporizes.

In the field, the best tactic is to squat or sit as low as you can; ideally on your foam pad or backpack, which will help insulate you from ground current. A group should be well spread out, so that a strike will not incapacitate everybody at once. Aboard a larger boat, avoid having the whole crew clustered in the cockpit.

Water is a good conductor, so don't swim or wade during a thunderstorm.

A relatively safe place is inside a car. The insulating value of the tires offers protection from ground current, and the metal shell conducts the energy of a direct strike around the occupants and into the ground. The metal shrouds and stays on a sailing vessel may have the same effect, provided there is a path to the water like a good grounding system or heavy cable led over the side from a shroud.

On a cliff, lightning current will follow the cliff face, especially where it's wet. Wet climbing ropes may also become conductors. Hollows and caves may seem attractive as shelter, but current can jump across the opening and include you in the path.

Because lightning can travel some distance (the longest documented lightning bolt exceeded 100 kilometers), you should evacuate hazardous areas as soon as thunder is heard. The rapid development of cumulonimbus clouds is an early warning, although orographic convection can cause lightning from a clear sky in dry climates. Lightning also can strike during snowfall in higher elevations.

NOTES:

NOTES:

Toxins

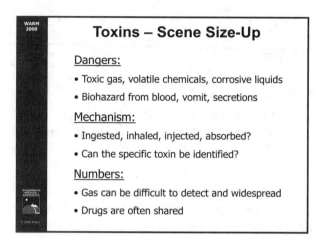

Toxins – Scene Size-Up

Dangers:
- Toxic gas, volatile chemicals, corrosive liquids
- Biohazard from blood, vomit, secretions

Mechanism:
- Ingested, inhaled, injected, absorbed?
- Can the specific toxin be identified?

Numbers:
- Gas can be difficult to detect and widespread
- Drugs are often shared

Toxic substances can produce systemic effects, local effects, or both. Toxins, like trauma, can cause simultaneous involvement of more than one body system. The cause and effect relationship may be fairly obvious, or quite confusing.

A toxin can also be an allergen causing a release of histamine in addition to its toxic effects. A hornet sting producing anaphylaxis is an example of a substance that can do both. Fortunately, a toxic reaction is not often mixed with allergy even though the type of exposure and symptoms may be similar.

Systemic toxins are those that affect the body as a whole. They may be ingested, injected, inhaled, or absorbed through the skin. Some common examples

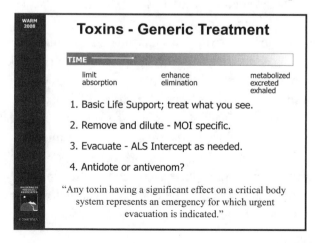

Toxins - Generic Treatment

TIME ⟶		
limit absorption	enhance elimination	metabolized excreted exhaled

1. Basic Life Support; treat what you see.

2. Remove and dilute - MOI specific.

3. Evacuate - ALS Intercept as needed.

4. Antidote or antivenom?

"Any toxin having a significant effect on a critical body system represents an emergency for which urgent evacuation is indicated."

include mushrooms, cobra venom, and carbon monoxide. These can represent an immediate threat to the function of the critical body systems.

Local toxins affect only the immediate area of contact. The toxin in a tarantula bite does not significantly affect critical body systems but may cause localized tissue swelling and pain. Some toxins have both systemic and local effects. An example would be an inhaled gas that irritates the respiratory system while being absorbed into the general circulation.

When you are not sure exactly what you're dealing with, base your initial treatment on the presenting signs and symptoms and the environmental conditions. In short, the generic response is to treat what you see. Support critical body systems. Treat anaphylaxis if you see it. Maintain body core temperature and hydration, and provide pain relief. Any toxin having a major effect on a critical body system represents an emergency for which urgent evacuation is indicated. While you should try to obtain as much information from the scene as possible, the investigation should not delay appropriate evacuation and life support, or increase the danger to rescuers.

INGESTED TOXINS

A brief review of anatomy reminds us that an ingested substance does not actually enter the body until it is absorbed by the lining of the digestive system. A glass marble swallowed by a child will not be absorbed, and will pass harmlessly through the gut. This is the goal for treatment of an ingested toxin, too.

We try to dilute the toxin and reduce its absorption using water and activated charcoal. At a dose of 25-50 grams orally, activated charcoal may bind the substances in the gut, helping to prevent absorption by the intestinal mucosa. Water will move the substance through the gut more quickly on its way to excretion.

Effective antidotes to toxins are not always available. Certainly their use is limited to cases where the toxin is known, such as certain drugs and plants. If possible, contact a poison control center (1-800-222-1222 in the US) or local medical facility for specific treatments. The availability of an antidote may influence your evacuation and destination. In any case, most toxins are excreted or metabolized by the body over hours or days.

DRUG OVERDOSE

You should know the risks associated with overdose of any drug that you carry in quantity. The likely source of a problem will be overuse of over-the-counter pain medication like acetaminophen and ibuprofen, or prescription narcotics like hydrocodone. Problems often occur when patients are confused about generic and trade names used for drugs. For example, a patient may take full doses of two different brands of pain reliever hoping for a better result, not realizing that both are brand names for the same acetaminophen. The effects of a mild unintentional overdose are usually limited to accentuated side effects like gastrointestinal (GI) upset or drowsiness. Discontinuing the medication usually solves the problem.

Intentional overdose is another matter. Even common over-the-counter medications like acetaminophen or iron tablets can be toxic in high doses. Immediate generic treatment followed by emergency evacuation is indicated. In narcotic or antihistamine overdose, the immediate threat to life will be respiratory failure due to loss of respiratory drive. Oxygen and PPV can be lifesaving.

FOOD POISONING

Food poisoning is another form of accidental toxic ingestion. The toxin is produced by bacteria such as staphylococci growing in poorly refrigerated food. The bacteria are usually destroyed by stomach acid,

but the toxin survives to be absorbed by the gut. Symptoms are usually limited to GI upset, including cramps, diarrhea, and vomiting. The disease is self-limiting, and the primary anticipated problem is shock from dehydration. Hydration is the primary treatment.

Food poisoning is differentiated from bacterial infection of the gut by the absence of fever or bloody or purulent diarrhea. Food poisoning is also very short-lived, usually resolving within 24 hours (an exception is Ciguatera). You should suspect infection in any gastrointestinal illness that lasts longer than that. A bacterial infection of the gut should be considered serious and aggressively treated with antibiotics or evacuation.

It may be impossible to distinguish a mild gastroenteritis caused by a viral infection from food poisoning because the signs and symptoms are often the same. Your primary clue will be the mechanism of injury. You should suspect food poisoning when a number of people who ate the same meal develop the same symptoms.

Ciguatera and scombroid are food-borne toxins worthy of special mention for the marine environment. Ciguatoxin is produced by a reef-dwelling dinoflagellate that is consumed by coral and other reef animals. It is concentrated up the food chain, reaching dangerous levels in larger predatory fish. It produces gastrointestinal symptoms as well as systemic neurologic symptoms such as numbness, tingling, cramping, and reversal of hot and cold sensation that may persist for weeks. Ciguatera toxin can be avoided by restricting the diet to fish smaller than a kilogram or so. It is not destroyed by cooking.

Scombroid toxin is a histamine-like substance produced by bacteria growing on the surface of dead fish in storage. Scombroid produces a histamine-like response including hives, itching, and flushed skin. It can be difficult to distinguish from an allergic reaction. Fortunately, the treatment is the same.

Symptoms developing after consumption of fish and shellfish should be treated like any other ingested toxin. Water and activated charcoal will help dilute and remove the toxin, minimizing absorption by the gut. Hives and itching can be effectively treated with an antihistamine like diphenhydramine or cimetadine. Persistent or severe neurological symptoms should be evacuated to medical care.

HIGH-RISK INGESTED TOXINS

If a toxin is known to be a high-risk problem, early evacuation to medical care is ideal. Examples include intentional acetaminophen overdose and symptoms developing after ingestion of an unknown mushroom species. In the remote setting where evacuation will be delayed or impossible, you should consider inducing vomiting. It is not completely effective, but performed quickly it can reduce the amount of toxin in the stomach.

The typical method is to administer syrup of ipecac, 15–30 cc orally followed by two cups of warm water. The patient will vomit within twenty minutes. After vomiting has ceased, give activated charcoal (25–50 grams) with water. This will help to keep the remaining toxin in the gut for excretion. Induction of vomiting is best done within first hour, but may be effective several hours post ingestion. Be sure that the patient is positioned to prevent airway obstruction.

You should not induce vomiting if the patient cannot protect his own airway. This treatment should not be used if the toxin is corrosive or a petroleum product. You must also be prepared to prevent dehydration and deal with thermoregulatory problems.

Vomiting should be considered a high-risk treatment. The need to carry ipecac as a treatment for toxic ingestion depends entirely on the population being served. It is something to consider if you care for young children or irresponsible adults.

TOPICAL EXPOSURE TO TOXINS

Clean the exposed area as you would for any skin wound. Irrigate copiously with water. Removal of some substances may require a different solvent capable of dissolving waxy or oily compounds. Alcohol, vinegar, and even WD-40 have found a place in initial treatment. Check with local medical facilities for recommendation on treating exposure to poisonous plants, preferably before the exposure occurs. Blisters should be left intact. Topical steroid creams may be helpful for superficial inflammation. Antibiotic ointment may help prevent infection.

Remember that the toxin may still be present on clothing and equipment that could come into contact with the patient or other members of the group. Examples of toxins that continue to spread on fingers and clothing include poison ivy (actually an allergen) and manchineel sap *(Hippomane mancinella)*. Clean your gear thoroughly to avoid perpetuating the problem.

HIGH-RISK TOPICAL EXPOSURE

As with large burns or abrasions, the surface area involved can lead to serious problems with even superficial injury. Anticipated problems in large surface area inflammation include dehydration, infection, and hypothermia. Any inflammatory process occupying more than about 10% body surface area should be considered high risk. Be alert to respiratory involvement that carries the anticipated problem of respiratory distress and failure.

INHALED TOXINS

Toxic inhalation can cause problems through two distinct mechanisms: inhaled substances can be absorbed through the respiratory system into the systemic circulation or cause direct respiratory system injury. Carbon monoxide poisoning from using a heater or stove inside a poorly vented snow cave is an example of the former, and chlorine gas is an example of the latter.

Carbon monoxide gas causes no direct respiratory system injury, but impairs oxygenation by displacing oxygen from receptor sites on hemoglobin molecules in red blood cells. Symptoms include headache, altered mental status, and nausea as the patient quietly asphyxiates. The problem may go unnoticed until it is too late. Like most inhaled toxins, the treatment is ventilation and fresh air. If instituted soon enough, there should be no lasting damage to critical body systems.

Direct injury can be caused by the inhalation of caustic substances. Chlorine gas directly damages the respiratory system. Symptoms include inflammation around the nose and mouth, coughing, wheezing, burning chest pain, and respiratory distress. Early recognition and treatment of respiratory distress is the key to survival. Identifying the causative agent in these cases is not as important as emergency field treatment and evacuation.

INJECTED TOXINS: BITES AND STINGS

Toxins used by organisms in the process of feeding or defense come in two basic types: neurotoxins and tissue toxins. Neurotoxins interfere with the function of the nervous system causing muscle spasm, paralysis, and altered sensation. In the rare cases of fatal neurotoxin envenomation, the cause of death is usually respiratory failure due to paralysis of the diaphragm and chest wall musculature.

Tissue toxins destroy body cells, causing inflammation, pain, and swelling. Damage is usually localized with distal ischemia and infection as anticipated problems. Severe envenomation can also produce systemic effects and multi-organ failure and volume shock.

Many organisms use a combination of tissue toxin and neurotoxin to subdue their prey. Antidotes are available to the toxins of some specific organisms and to some groups of similar species. Before traveling become knowledgeable about local toxic species and the availability and location of antivenoms.

The vast majority of stings and bites are no more significant than the minimal discomfort that they cause. The few that are significant are easily identified by severe pain, swelling, or the progression of neurological symptoms. The important principle of field treatment for significant envenomation is to provide good basic life support while moving toward the appropriate definitive medical care. The identification of the specific species encountered can be valuable in planning treatment if medical facilities are accessible, but should not delay evacuation.

MARINE TOXINS

In the marine environment, toxins are most commonly infiltrated by spines or injected by nematocysts. They range in potency from the merely annoying to the rapidly fatal. Again, the recognition of species is not as important as the recognition and treatment of a critical system problem.

Spiny Injury – Spines are used for defense and some are coated with toxins. Examples include stingrays, scorpion fish, catfish, and some sea urchins. The species found in waters around North America generally produce only the localized pain and swelling of tissue toxins. In Indo-Pacific waters the organisms can be more dangerous carrying significant neurotoxic effects as well *(e.g., cone shell)*.

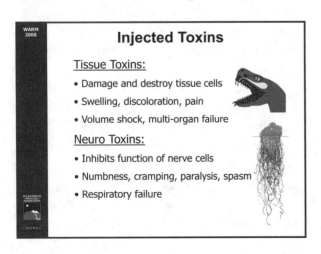

Injected Toxins

Tissue Toxins:
• Damage and destroy tissue cells
• Swelling, discoloration, pain
• Volume shock, multi-organ failure

Neuro Toxins:
• Inhibits function of nerve cells
• Numbness, cramping, paralysis, spasm
• Respiratory failure

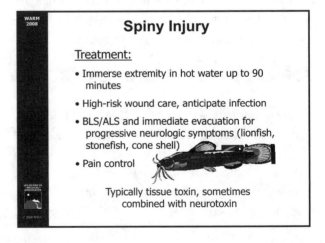

Spiny Injury

Treatment:
• Immerse extremity in hot water up to 90 minutes
• High-risk wound care, anticipate infection
• BLS/ALS and immediate evacuation for progressive neurologic symptoms (lionfish, stonefish, cone shell)
• Pain control

Typically tissue toxin, sometimes combined with neurotoxin

The sting of a poisonous ray, urchin, or fish is easy to distinguish from a non-toxic puncture. The pain caused by the wound itself is minimal compared to the quickly increasing discomfort caused by the toxin, which may possess both tissue toxic and neurotoxic characteristics. The barbed stinger or spine will often remain in the wound. Because the spine may be coated with a sheath of tissue that contaminates the wound, infection is likely. Treatment includes removing the spine or stinger and aggressive wound debridement.

Many types of spiny toxins are inactivated by heat. Immerse the affected part in water as hot as the patient can tolerate until pain is relieved. Often this will be within a few minutes, but treatment may need to be continued for an hour or more.

Nematocyst Stings – Nematocysts are structures in the stinging parts of jellyfish, corals, and anemones, which fire something resembling a microscopic harpoon when touched. These harpoons then inject a potent neurotoxin into the skin. Individually the amount of toxin is miniscule, but the toxin load can be considerable when the patient contacts thousands of nematocysts at once. Of particular concern are stings from the Indo-Pacific box jellyfish (Chironex fleckeri) due to the high-potency of the venom and the Portuguese man-of-war due to the potential for large surface area exposure.

The general field treatment for stinging jellyfish includes removing tentacles by flushing with seawater and picking off any remaining tentacles with forceps or gloved fingers. Seawater is considered preferable to fresh water because the osmotic difference of fresh water may stimulate more nematocysts to fire. Flushing and soaking the skin with vinegar will inactivate the nematocysts of some species and is specifically recommended for box jellyfish, fireworm, and sponge stings. Ice applications may help relieve the pain. The use of alcohol, meat tenderizer, urine, or other chemicals to flush the skin is not helpful, and possibly harmful.

Persistent skin inflammation can be treated for several days with twice daily applications of a steroid cream or ointment *(e.g., hydrocortisone)*. Antihistamines may also help because a local allergic reaction may be part of the patient's discomfort. As with any open wound, infection is an anticipated problem.

Systemic effects from large or potent exposure to nematocyst-borne neurotoxins include pain, spasm, and cramping. An exposure occupying more than 50% of a limb should be considered potentially serious with anticipated systemic neurotoxic effects. Truly life-threatening symptoms are generally limited to Portuguese man-of-war and the Indo-Pacific box jellyfish. Medical follow-up is recommended for any exposure that produces significant systemic symptoms.

The box jellyfish venom can produce cardiac arrhythmia, respiratory paralysis, and a dangerous elevation of blood pressure. For this reason, antivenom to this toxin is carried and administered in the field by rescue personnel in high-incidence areas of Australia and Southeast Asia. BLS and immediate evacuation are indicated. Consult local authorities about the area you plan to operate in.

There is no antivenom for the Portuguese man-of-war. Fortunately, fatalities from exposure are very rare. Symptoms include severe burning sensations and skin redness that tends to disappear within an hour. Initial treatment includes only flushing with water, removal of tentacles, and treatment for pain. In the case of Portuguese man-of-war, vinegar is not recommended.

More significant exposure can cause muscle

WARM 2008

Nematocyst Injury

Treatment:

• Rinse with salt water, remove tentacles

• Vinegar soaks (most species)

• General wound care, topical corticosteroids

• BLS/ALS and immediate evacuation for progressive neurologic symptoms (box jelly, man-of-war)

• Pain control

Typically neurotoxic effects with skin inflammation

cramping, temporary numbness and weakness in the area, and lymph node swelling. Allergic reactions are uncommon, but the practitioner should be alert to the signs and symptoms of anaphylaxis mixed with the toxic effects. Any persistent or severe symptoms require follow-up medical care.

SNAKEBITE

In North America there are two types of poisonous snakes: pit vipers and coral snakes. The pit vipers include rattlesnakes, copperheads, and cottonmouths. Pit viper venom is primarily a tissue toxin that causes local swelling and tissue damage. Systemic effects include problems with blood coagulation and shock caused by leakage of fluid from the circulatory system into the interstitial space (between the cells in body tissues). Some pit viper venom, notably the Mojave rattlesnake, also contains a systemic neurotoxin. The degree of systemic effect depends on the dose injected and the size and general health of the patient. Fatalities in North America are extremely rare.

The specific and ideal treatment for poisonous snakebite is antivenom. Evacuation to medical care should be started without delay by the fastest means available. Walking your patient out may be the quickest way to go, and this is fine unless prevented by severe symptoms. If possible, alert the receiving facility to expect your patient so that antivenom can be acquired and prepared.

The use of antivenom is restricted to the hospital because it can cause life-threatening allergic reactions in rare cases. It is also extremely expensive and needs to be prepared carefully prior to use. It is most effective in the first four hours, but can be given up to several days following the bite and still have some benefit.

Pit viper antivenom is the same for all of the members of that family of snakes. It is not necessary to know the difference between a rattlesnake, copperhead, or cottonmouth. The presence of fang marks is enough.

Splinting the bitten extremity may help reduce pain and tissue damage, but it is an unproven treatment and should not delay evacuation. If ALS is easily available, IV hydration with isotonic saline should be initiated. Do not apply ice or arterial or venous tourniquets. Do not apply suction or incise the wound. Suction devices, even the more modern versions, have been shown to be ineffective and possibly harmful.

In anticipation of swelling, remove constricting items such as rings, bracelets, and tight clothing to prevent ischemia. Closely monitor any splint. If

---

Pit Vipers (Crotalines)

Rattlesnake/Copperhead/Cottonmouth:

• Triangular head

• Heat sensing "pits"

• Inject venom through fangs

• Mostly tissue toxic

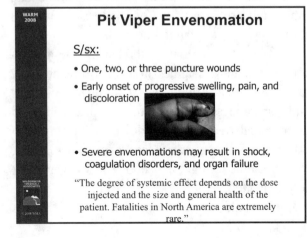

Pit Viper Envenomation

S/sx:

• One, two, or three puncture wounds

• Early onset of progressive swelling, pain, and discoloration

• Severe envenomations may result in shock, coagulation disorders, and organ failure

"The degree of systemic effect depends on the dose injected and the size and general health of the patient. Fatalities in North America are extremely rare."

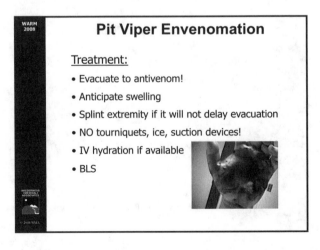

Pit Viper Envenomation

Treatment:

• Evacuate to antivenom!

• Anticipate swelling

• Splint extremity if it will not delay evacuation

• NO tourniquets, ice, suction devices!

• IV hydration if available

• BLS

you can, mark the progression of swelling up the extremity. Make a line and write the time on the skin with a pen. This information will be helpful in the decision to use antivenom, and in deciding how much will be necessary.

The amount of venom injected varies with the size and condition of the snake. Symptoms can range from mild to severe. A small number of strikes are dry bites where no venom is injected at all. This is worth remembering if emergency evacuation will be a high-risk operation. In these situations, medical care may be delayed if no symptoms develop or the swelling remains localized and progression stops within three hours.

Coral snake venom is neurotoxic. The fangs of the coral snake are quite small. The snake will have to chew its way into your skin to successfully inject venom. It requires handling of the snake to be bitten. The victims are usually children or intoxicated teenage males. The venom's effects may be delayed for several hours.

Symptoms of coral snake bite include tingling of the extremity, possibly progressing to the whole body. Fatalities, due to respiratory failure, are also

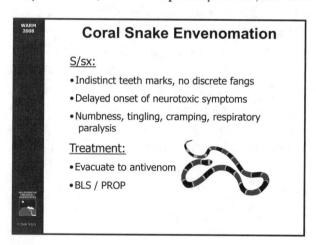

Coral Snake Envenomation

WARM 2008

S/sx:

- Indistinct teeth marks, no discrete fangs
- Delayed onset of neurotoxic symptoms
- Numbness, tingling, cramping, respiratory paralysis

Treatment:

- Evacuate to antivenom
- BLS / PROP

rare. The specific treatment is coral snake antivenom. Fortunately, a coral snake is easily distinguished from a pit viper.

In parts of the world outside of North America, fang-bearing snakes possess more destructive forms of venom. A lymphatic compression bandage is sometimes employed in the field treatment of

envenomation known to involve potent neurotoxins. It is worth research into the types of snakes, recommended treatments, and location of antivenom for the region in which you will be traveling. You may find, for example, that the nearest antivenin for the Fer de Lance in Trinidad is actually in Miami. Check before you need it.

INSECTS AND ARACHNIDS

Insect and arachnid venom is injected by a stinger or specialized mouthparts as the animal attempts to defend itself or warn you away from a nest. It is meant to hurt, and it usually does. This is typical of wasps, fire ants, spiders, and scorpions.

More commonly, your skin reacts to the irritation of substances used by a feeding insect to prevent clotting of your blood. Many of them also inject a local anesthetic to reduce the pain caused by the bite, at least for as long as they're feeding. Examples of these insects include black flies, moose flies, mosquitoes, and no-see-ums.

Local reaction to toxins can be severe, but involve only the extremity or immediate area of the bite or sting. There may be some degree of ASR that must be distinguished from systemic effects. Local reactions are treated for comfort. Use cool soaks, elevation, and rest. Aspirin, ibuprofen, or other anti-inflammatory pain medications will help, as will diphenhydramine or other antihistamines.

Toxin load is the term applied to the cumulative effects of multiple stings or bites. The effects can be immediate as with a large number of bee stings, or delayed up to 24 hours. Delayed reactions are common in black fly country in the spring and early summer. Symptoms include fever, fatigue, headache, and nausea. This is not an allergic reaction if the generalized swelling, respiratory distress, and other signs of anaphylaxis are absent.

Toxin load is usually not a major critical system problem. Observe for 24 hours. Give aspirin, ibuprofen, or other anti-inflammatory pain reliever for comfort. Watch for signs of infection at the site of insect bites. Keep the patient well hydrated and protected from excessive cooling or heating.

Black Widow – The black widow spider *(Latrodectus mactans)*, found in the warmer parts of the United States and further south, uses a potent neurotoxin to immobilize prey and as a defense mechanism. This spider prefers dark and quiet places to feed and nest. People are bitten most often when reaching into confined spaces or sitting on an outhouse seat. The bite itself is mildly uncomfortable or painless.

The systemic symptoms of black widow envenomation include muscle cramping (especially in the abdomen), severe pain, numbness, and tingling. The development of these symptoms shortly after crawling around likely habitat should raise the suspicion of a black widow bite. Treatment includes evacuation to medical care because your patient may require critical system support and medication to reduce muscle spasm. Antivenin is available, but may carry more risk than the venom itself. Symptoms usually resolve over several days. In spite of its ominous name, death from the bite of a black widow is rare.

Brown Recluse – The brown recluse is a large spider found in the south central United States that injects a long-acting tissue toxin causing localized tissue inflammation and necrosis. The initial bite may go unnoticed, with a pustule developing several days later. This is often mistaken for an infection caused by a splinter or other foreign body. It does not respond to incision and drainage or to antibiotics. Although many of these envenomations resolve uneventfully, the lesion can continue to progress over days and weeks to involve a large area of tissue destruction that may become secondarily infected. A suspected brown recluse bite should be referred to a surgeon.

Centroidies – Most scorpion stings are described as similar to or a bit worse than your average wasp. Most annoying in North America is the Centroidies excilicauda that employs a potent neurotoxin. Pain may last for hours or days. There is no specific field treatment beyond pain medication. Ice is not indicated. Significant systemic symptoms are rare and include agitation and respiratory paralysis; these should prompt an evacuation to medical care. An antivenin is available, but it is a high-risk treatment due to the incidence of serum sickness and anaphylaxis. No fatalities from Centroidies stings have been reported in the United States.

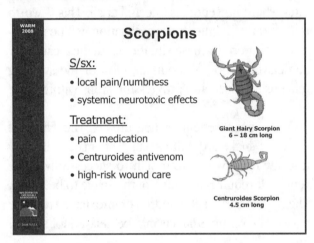

Ticks – The saliva of some species of ticks contains a neurotoxin capable of causing symptoms in humans, most commonly in children. Tick paralysis can develop after four or more days of attachment and is characterized by numbness and paralysis progressing up the legs and arms. The patient may exhibit ataxia, restless, or irritability. The diagnosis is suspected by finding an engorged tick and confirmed by rapid improvement following its removal.

Tick paralysis is rare. Ticks are more commonly implicated as vectors of disease (discussed in the next chapter). Prevention of tick paralysis and tick-borne disease depends on avoiding bites and early removal of attached ticks.

CASE STUDY: TOXINS

S: An 18-year-old male on a spring break canoe trip on Lake Powell was bitten on the left forearm by a four-foot snake that he was attempting to capture and bring back to camp. In the ensuing confusion, the snake escaped. The man was unable to describe it other than being dark in color and very fast. He complained of pain in the mid left forearm, and of feeling very faint.

It was early evening, the sky was clear, and the temperature was about 20°C The camp was located approximately seven miles from the marina at Bullfrog. In spite of a stiff headwind on the lake, the patient was carried to a canoe for evacuation to the marina. Unfortunately, the paddlers were also intoxicated and became lost in the darkness. They returned to camp two hours later, unsure of where they had been.

The patient was reevaluated by a Wilderness First Responder who had not been drinking. The patient, now calm and alert, reported no allergies and was not taking any medication. He had no past history of significant medical problems and had eaten dinner four hours ago, which included a six-pack of beer. There was no other recent trauma or illness.

O: The patient was awake but subdued, with normal mental status. He had two small puncture wounds on his left forearm. There was minimal swelling extending seven centimeters proximal to the bite, but no discoloration. The area was mildly tender to the touch. Distal CSM was intact. There were no other injuries. Vital Signs at 10:15 p.m. were —BP: unavailable, P: 80, R: 16, T: appears normal, Skin: W/D/P. C: Awake and oriented.

A: 1. Pit viper bite
        A': local and systemic effects of the toxin
    2. Dark, windy
        A': Hazardous evacuation

P: 1. Rings and watch removed from the arm. Continued monitoring
    2. Keep overnight in camp, evacuate in daylight

Discussion: The decision to stay in camp was based on the low risk of further serious problems from the snakebite and the high risk of waterborne evacuation in the dark. Proceeding with evacuation in the morning was appropriate, even though symptoms had not progressed. Problems with blood coagulation and compartment syndrome can develop later and should be monitored. A bite is also considered a high-risk wound.

NOTES:

Arthropod Disease Vectors

The phylum Arthropoda includes insects, spiders, crustaceans and others comprising over 80% of known animal species. Since many of them feed on humans, they are a significant mechanism for the transmission of disease. Some arthropods merely transmit viruses or bacteria from person to person. Others serve as a host for one stage of the parasite life-cycle with humans hosting another. In either case, illness is often the result.

TICKS

Ticks are a problem as a vector for diseases like Lyme disease, Colorado tick fever, ehrlichiosis, babesiosis, and Rocky Mountain spotted fever. Fortunately for the wilderness medical practitioner, most of these conditions only manifest themselves many days to weeks after exposure. Unfortunately for the patient and his doctor, these present with a constellation of confusing symptoms making a definitive diagnosis difficult. The primary work of the practitioner in the field is prevention and education.

Inform your teammates or expedition members of the risks involved in feeding ticks. Instruct them to wear long sleeved shirt with long pants tucked into high socks, and a bandanna high on the neck under a

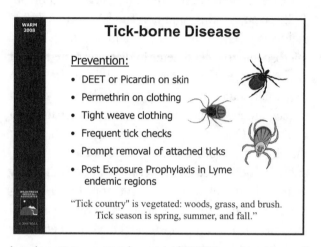

Tick-borne Disease

Prevention:

- DEET or Picardin on skin
- Permethrin on clothing
- Tight weave clothing
- Frequent tick checks
- Prompt removal of attached ticks
- Post Exposure Prophylaxis in Lyme endemic regions

"Tick country" is vegetated: woods, grass, and brush. Tick season is spring, summer, and fall."

low hat. Encourage the use of DEET on the skin and pemethrin on clothing, especially around cuff and neck openings. By following these recommendations, your team members may look silly, but such precautions will substantially reduce the chance of feeding a tick and acquiring a tick borne disease.

It is also important to frequently check for ticks on your skin and clothing. They usually will crawl around for a while before settling in to feed. Frequent inspections will get rid of most of them before they attach.

Ticks that are attached can be most safely removed by grasping them at the skin surface and gently pulling them off with tweezers. Sometimes, the mouthparts will break off and be left in the skin. Try to scrape these out with a sharp blade or needle.

The patient should not attempt removal by burning the tick, or suffocating or poisoning it with Vaseline, alcohol, gasoline, or mineral oil. These tactics may cause the tick to regurgitate infectious material into the bite. Do not handle the tick without gloves or other protection.

Prompt removal of ticks can also help reduce the transmission of disease. Lyme disease, for example, is not effectively transmitted until the tick has been in place for a day or so. Rocky Mountain spotted fever can

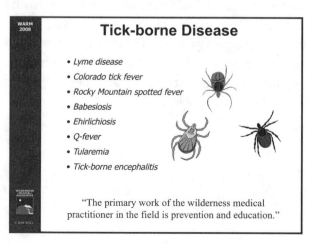

Tick-borne Disease

- Lyme disease
- Colorado tick fever
- Rocky Mountain spotted fever
- Babesiosis
- Ehirlichiosis
- Q-fever
- Tularemia
- Tick-borne encephalitis

"The primary work of the wilderness medical practitioner in the field is prevention and education."

be transmitted in just a few hours. In regions where Lyme disease is endemic, medical practitioners will often prescribe a single dose treatment of doxycycline or other antibiotic to patients who have suffered a prolonged tick attachment.

Tick country is vegetated: woods, grass, and brush. Tick season is spring, summer, and fall. Adult ticks are eight-legged arthropods ranging in size from nearly microscopic to a centimeter in diameter. The ticks of greatest concern, for Lyme disease at least, are two to four millimeters in diameter, and before they begin to feed are easily recognized as a foreign creature on your skin. Once attached and engorged with blood, they look more like a wart, mole, or other skin part, and may be missed by someone who doesn't know your body as well as you do. The appearance of flu-like symptoms, severe headaches, fever, rash, and muscular aches and pains several days to weeks after a confirmed long-term tick attachment or travel in a tick infested area is worth bringing to the attention of a medical practitioner.

MOSQUITOES

The list of diseases transmitted by mosquitoes includes malaria, filiariasis, West Nile virus, equine encephalitis, and a host of others. The key to avoiding these infections is to avoid being a host to mosquitoes. Like ticks, they can be deterred by insect repellent and tight-weave clothing. Unlike ticks, they can transmit disease in less than a minute.

Prophylactic medication with malarone or doxycycline can help prevent malaria infection. However, some diseases like filarisis have no definitive cure and no effective prophylactic medication. The fewer mosquitoes you feed, the less your chance of becoming ill.

The best insect repellents currently available include DEET, pemethrin, and picardin. DEET and pemethrin are both extensively studied and are considered safe and effective. DEET can be used on the exposed skin of hands, ankles, and the face. There is no advantage to using a formulation greater than 35% DEET. Pemethrin is recommended for clothing and has been shown to remain effective after 20 or more washings.

FLEAS AND LICE

Only about 5% of a given flea population is actively feeding on blood. The rest are various stages of development as eggs, pupae and larvae. Adult fleas can hibernate for up to two years waiting for a blood meal.

The worst place to sleep is on that old mattress in the trekking hut that was last occupied six weeks ago. The eggs, pupae, and larvae have matured and are waiting for you. Only a few of them need to be carrying the bacteria Yersinia pestis to give you bubonic plague. Fleas can be killed or deterred by insect repellents and insecticides. Your own sleeping bag, frequently washed, is another good defense.

Lice are easily transmitted between people sharing clothing and furniture. The adults are easily killed with pemethrin or malathione. Reapplication may be necessary in ten days to kill the newly hatched larvae. In the absence of pemethrin shampoo, lice can also be smothered with a layer of any viscous substance like Vaseline or mayonnaise. It may not be pretty, but it can solve your problem!

WARM 2008

Mosquito-borne Disease

Prevention:

- DEET or Picardin on skin
- Permethrin on clothing
- Tight weave clothing
- Avoid feeding time
- Pre or post exposure prophylaxis in Malaria endemic regions*

* See www.cdc.gov

Section V

Backcountry Medicine

An Approach to Illness

The nonspecific symptoms of many illnesses can generate a long list of possible diagnoses. Even in the emergency department, it can be difficult to figure out exactly what you're dealing with. In the backcountry it can be impossible. Our working diagnosis may remain as generic as "serious," "not serious," or "I don't know."

There is little value in working through lists of symptoms and descriptions of diseases just so you can put a name on your patient's problem. The laboratory and x-ray aren't available to confirm your suspicions anyway. Your primary job in dealing with illness is to keep your patient safe, comfortable, and well hydrated and to watch for the development of anything serious.

As you evaluate an illness, beware of focusing too much attention on isolated signs or symptoms. Consider vital signs in the context of the patient's behavior. For example, you should worry much more about a confused and lethargic person with a temperature of 37° C, than an active and oriented patient with a fever of 40° C.

Your initial evaluation of an ill patient is essentially the same as that for trauma. Observe and measure the function of the three critical systems to detect on-going or anticipated problems. A patient with a cough, for example, may have a respiratory infection with the anticipated problem of respiratory distress. A complaint of diarrhea carries the anticipated problem of dehydration and shock. The likelihood of respiratory distress, shock, or other critical system problem determines the severity of the illness.

It is also worth remembering that a healthy person willingly takes in food and fluid, and produces urine and feces in more or less proportional amounts. Such people are interested in their surroundings and know who they are and what they're doing. They will freely move, dress, and protect themselves from the environment.

A patient who is ill but basically sound may be uncomfortable but will continue to eat and drink and function more or less normally. These patients are not particularly worrisome. It is when your patient stops eating and drinking, loses interest in her surroundings, and is unable to take care of herself that you should consider the situation serious. This is the time to perform BLS functions and plan an evacuation, regardless of the diagnosis.

Pain is another complaint worth careful investigation. The location and character will sometimes lead you to a more specific diagnosis. Any pain that seems severe and out of proportion to what you see wrong should be taken as a sign of a potentially serious problem.

So, your initial assessment of the ill patient begins with an evaluation of the circulatory, respiratory, and nervous systems looking for existing or anticipated problems. Your history evaluates the patient's regular functions of food and fluid intake, and the output of urine and feces. Finally, the examiner investigates any complaint of pain. This process should detect the presence of any serious condition, guide your physical exam, and lead you toward a more specific assessment and plan.

WARM 2008

An Approach to Illness

- Critical System Problem?
- Ins and outs?
- Pain?
- Mental Status?
- Serious, Not Serious or I Don't Know?

"Even in the emergency department, it can be difficult to figure out exactly what you're dealing with. Our working diagnosis may remain as generic as *serious*, *not serious*, or *I don't know.*"

NOTES:

Treating Pain

26

Pain has a purpose: to keep us from damaging ourselves. But once the damage is done pain becomes a management problem. It is a natural and appropriate reaction for you to want to relieve someone's suffering, especially if you are the caregiver.

The most effective form of pain relief is to correct the cause. Reduce the dislocation, loosen the splint, drain the abscess, or rehydrate the dried out hiker with the headache. Secondary swelling can be reduced with elevation and cooling. Unstable injuries are less painful when effectively stabilized. Acute partial-thickness burns are less painful when occlusive dressings are applied. Ask the patient what feels better, and help him to achieve it.

Sometimes, however, definitive field treatment is not possible or does not completely fix the problem. The pain remains. We are left to treat the pain as a symptom, being fully aware that the original problem has not been solved.

Medications for pain come in three basic forms: NSAIDs, other non-narcotic analgesics, and narcotics. NSAIDs are the non-steroidal anti-inflammatory drugs such as aspirin, ibuprofen, and naproxen sodium. These drugs work by inhibiting the action of some of the chemical mediators of inflammation and pain at the site of injury. The result is fewer pain impulses being transmitted from the injury to the brain. The various NSAIDs work in slightly different ways, but all work to reduce pain, fever, and inflammation. Ibuprofen is a good example, and very effective in therapeutic doses of 600–800 mg every eight hours for an adult.

Non-steroidal drugs like ibuprofen do not significantly affect brain function. The patient remains awake and functional, distinct advantages in a hazardous setting. NSAIDs are the first line medication for the treatment of pain, inflammation, and fever in most backcountry situations. Just be sure to maintain adequate hydration to prevent kidney damage when using NSAIDs.

The primary side effects of NSAIDs include stomach irritation and increased bleeding. These drugs may not be a good choice for someone with nausea from sea sickness, and certainly are not for a patient where life-threatening bleeding is an anticipated problem. A better non-narcotic analgesic for these patients would be acetaminophen. Like the NSAIDs, acetaminophen provides good pain relief and reduction of fever. Unlike the NSAIDs, it tends not to cause stomach upset or increased bleeding. Acetaminophen, however, does not have significant anti-inflammatory effects and will not help reduce swelling or tissue damage caused by inflammation.

Narcotics work on pain by reducing the brain's ability to receive pain impulses from the site of injury. Unfortunately, narcotics depress other brain function as well. Side effects include increased reaction time, drowsiness, and depressed respiratory drive. Narcotics also reduce gut motility, causing constipation. In some situations, these side effects may be unacceptable.

In spite of these disadvantages, narcotics are best for moderate to severe pain where the patient can be monitored and protected. In most of the world, narcotics are available only by prescription and should

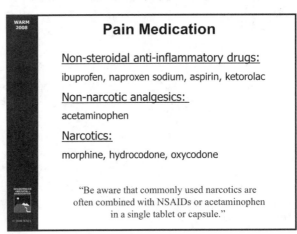

WARM 2008

Pain Medication

<u>Non-steroidal anti-inflammatory drugs:</u>
ibuprofen, naproxen sodium, aspirin, ketorolac

<u>Non-narcotic analgesics:</u>
acetaminophen

<u>Narcotics:</u>
morphine, hydrocodone, oxycodone

"Be aware that commonly used narcotics are often combined with NSAIDs or acetaminophen in a single tablet or capsule."

©2008 WMA

be used under the guidance of a medical practitioner. For backcountry use, narcotics can be administered by routes that do not require injection. Morphine can be given as a tablet. Fentanyl can be given in the form of an oral lollipop or skin patch.

Be aware that commonly used narcotics are often combined with NSAIDs or acetaminophen in a single tablet or capsule. Vicodin is a combination of hydrocodone and acetaminophen. Vicoprofen is hydrocodone combined with ibuprofen. Percocet is oxycodone combined with acetaminophen. The combinations are numerous and the names are rarely helpful. To avoid an overdose, be sure that you know what you are dispensing and what your patient is already using.

NOTES:

Abdominal Pain

27

The differential diagnosis for abdominal pain is extensive. Making a specific diagnosis can be a challenge for experienced clinicians, even when using laboratory data and sophisticated imaging equipment. This is a good time for the wilderness medical practitioner to base treatment and evacuation decisions on a generic assessment. Is the pain the symptom of a condition that is serious or not serious? Because the treatment of a serious intra-abdominal problem will require hospital and surgical care anyway, the specific diagnosis can usually wait.

THE ABDOMEN

For field purposes, we can consider the contents and structure of the abdomen to consist of four major components: hollow organs, solid organs, the peritoneal lining, and the muscular abdominal wall. Hollow structures like the stomach, intestines, and gall bladder are muscular organs that excrete and move fluids and food through the digestive system by rhythmic muscle contractions called *peristalsis*. The ureters and urinary bladder are of similar structure and function to contain and excrete urine.

Solid organs within the abdomen have a variety of functions and associated diseases, but we worry most about their potential for rupture in abdominal trauma. The liver, spleen, pancreas, and kidneys are part of the body core and are richly supplied with blood. These structures can fracture on impact, and bleeding can be severe. The abdomen offers enough potential space for blood loss to allow for life-threatening volume shock.

The peritoneum is the membrane that lines all of the abdominal organs and the abdominal wall. It is easily irritated by bacteria, blood, and digestive fluids that have leaked into the abdominal cavity. Because the peritoneum represents a surface area greater than

that of your patient's skin, it can lose a large volume of fluid in a short period of time when it becomes inflamed. Much like a large surface area burn, extensive peritonitis will result in volume shock.

The muscular wall of the abdomen lies outside of the peritoneum, and therefore it is not within the abdominal cavity. These skeletal muscles provide protection and support for the abdominal contents. They contract in response to both the commands associated with voluntary movement and the involuntary need for abdominal protection. The muscles themselves can also be a source of pain that can be difficult to distinguish from intra-abdominal problems.

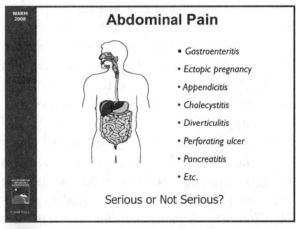

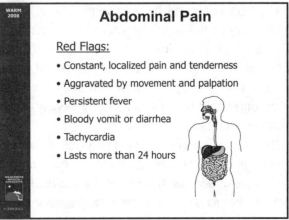

The assessment of abdominal pain requires a basic understanding of the structure, function, and nerve supply of the abdominal organs. The nerve cells in hollow organs transmit pain sensations primarily when stretched, like when your stomach is distended by a big meal. Stretching of a hollow organ stimulates muscular contraction, causing the pain of distention to temporarily become worse. We usually call this a cramp.

It is also useful to note that the nerve supply to the gut is general in nature. The esophagus, stomach, and upper small intestine are supplied by sensory nerves exiting the spinal cord at the level of the epigastrum (upper abdomen). The small intestine and very proximal large intestine is supplied by nerves exiting at the level of the umbilicus (navel). The colon and rectum (large intestine) is enervated at the level of the lower abdomen and pelvis. The pain of a distended hollow organ tends to be poorly localized at the general level of enervation, rather than identified as a specific spot.

Because peristalsis increases the pain in waves, the discomfort tends to be intermittent. If the problem is well contained within the gut, the chief complaint remains as intermittent, crampy, poorly localized abdominal pain. The mechanism is usually gas, fluid, and spasm created by a viral illness, food intolerance, or constipation.

The patient with mild abdominal pain may tighten the abdominal wall muscles in response to the pressure of your abdominal palpation, but can voluntarily relax them when encouraged to do so. This is known as *voluntary guarding*. Any tenderness elicited on exam will be nonspecific and relatively mild. Bowel sounds will be normal to hyperactive. This kind of abdominal pain is usually associated with mild conditions that are well contained within the gut, not affecting the abdominal cavity itself. The symptoms might be unpleasant but generally do not indicate a serious problem.

If the condition within the gut progresses to a more serious problem, you may begin to see the signs and symptoms of peritoneal irritation. Unlike the hollow organs, the peritoneum is specifically enervated like your skin surface. An inflamed peritoneum causes localized pain aggravated by movement as the inflamed membranes rub against each other.

APPENDICITIS AND OTHER HOLLOW ORGAN PROBLEMS

In a textbook case of appendicitis, the problem begins with obstruction. The appendix is a hollow organ connected to the large intestine in the lower right quadrant of the abdomen. Obstruction of the appendix ultimately leads to infection and swelling. The early symptoms are often the generalized, crampy discomfort typical of intestinal distention. Because the appendix and first few centimeters of the large intestine are actually enervated with the small intestine, the pain is felt around the umbilicus. It would be impossible to distinguish this from mild gas pains, and you would not label it as serious.

As the infection progresses, the swollen and inflamed appendix will begin to irritate the peritoneal lining of the intestine and abdomen. The symptoms will begin to change from generalized periumbilical cramping to localized constant pain in the right lower quadrant. Abdominal wall muscle spasm will cause involuntary guarding as the body protects the abdominal contents from movement. Palpation will elicit tenderness that tends to be specific to the problem area. Jostling or walking the patient will produce pain in the same location. Peristalsis will slow or stop, and bowel sounds will diminish dramatically. These are called peritoneal signs, and indicate a serious problem within the abdomen.

If the appendicitis is allowed to progress, the organ may burst spilling digestive enzymes and pus into the abdominal cavity and peritoneal lining. Pain will be severe, constant, and will spread throughout the abdomen. Shock and death are often the result.

The key to early recognition of appendicitis is the change in character of the pain from the crampy and generalized pain of hollow organ distention to the constant and localized pain of peritoneal inflammation. Other less specific signs and symptoms like fever, diarrhea, vomiting, and tachycardia all add to your concern.

The same progression of signs and symptoms can occur with other hollow organ problems like cholecystitis, ectopic pregnancy, bowel obstruction, and an infected diverticulum. It is not necessary to know exactly what you're dealing with to know that it needs a surgeon and an operating room. Peritoneal signs indicate a serious abdominal problem regardless of the location or cause.

OTHER ABDOMINAL PROBLEMS

Solid organ rupture and bleeding can also cause irritation of the peritoneal lining. The wilderness medical practitioner should be alert to the development of peritoneal signs following significant blunt trauma to the abdomen. With constant pain and localized tenderness, volume shock from internal bleeding is the anticipated problem.

Of course, a similar type of pain can be caused by muscle contusion or strain of the abdominal wall. This may not be associated with any internal organs and is not serious, but it can be difficult to distinguish from peritoneal irritation. This type of pain will usually be relieved by rest and made worse specifically by use of the injured muscles.

Even if the abdominal pain itself is not identified as serious, an illness with vomiting and diarrhea may lead you to anticipate volume shock from dehydration. The presence of blood or pus in the stool or vomit indicates a serious infection. If rehydration and definitive treatment in the field is not possible, evacuation is indicated even if surgery is not. The potential for dehydration and the presence of an infection in the gut are included in the red flags for abdominal pain.

TREATMENT OF ABDOMINAL PAIN

Red flags mean evacuation. You should continue to monitor the patient during transport and note any changes in condition. In the long-term care setting, abdominal pain or the accompanying red flags may resolve, revealing the problem to be less serious.

In this case, it is better to cancel or slow down an evacuation in progress rather that start one too late.

If the evacuation will exceed two hours or so, give fluids and calories to make up for normal and abnormal losses. This should be restricted to water, rehydration solutions, and easily absorbed simple sugars. Oral pain medication should be restricted to acetaminophen because other anti-inflammatory drugs can irritate the gut. If narcotics are available, injectable medication is preferred. Pain medication should not be withheld in the belief that it will mask serious symptoms or inhibit diagnosis in the emergency room.

Abdominal pain labeled as not serious can be treated symptomatically with due attention to hydration and calories. The patient should not take NSAIDs to avoid further irritating the gut. Acetaminophen would be a better choice. Gut soothers like bismuth subsalicylate and antacids are generally safe. Food should be restricted to easily digested carbohydrates and sugars. Vomiting and diarrhea can be treated with anti-emetics like meclizine or diphenhydramine and with mild narcotic anti-spasmotics like loprimide provided there are no signs of bacterial infection. The patient should be frequently monitored for the development of peritoneal signs or dehydration.

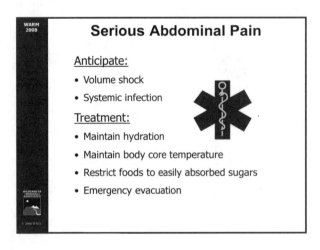

Serious Abdominal Pain

Anticipate:
- Volume shock
- Systemic infection

Treatment:
- Maintain hydration
- Maintain body core temperature
- Restrict foods to easily absorbed sugars
- Emergency evacuation

NOTES:

Chest Pain

28

As with the abdomen, there are a number of possible causes of chest pain. Again, our diagnosis is often limited to the generic assessment: serious or not serious. With a history of significant trauma, any persistent chest pain should be considered serious. In the absence of trauma, the type of chest pain that we most worry about is the pain of myocardial ischemia.

The mechanism may be an acute clot or spasm in a coronary artery or it may be a chronic coronary artery constriction that prevents adequate blood flow to the heart muscle when oxygen demand is increased. Either way, the heart muscle is ischemic and not getting enough oxygen. If the condition persists, infarction will result.

If the area of the heart that is ischemic includes a major branch of the electrical conduction system, a cardiac arrhythmia may develop. Whether you refer to it as myocardial ischemia or heart attack, it is a major circulatory system problem with the anticipated problem of cardiogenic shock and death.

The pain of myocardial ischemia can present in a variety of ways: from the classic sub-sternal pain radiating to the jaw and left arm, to back or abdominal pain. The patient may also experience shortness of breath, sweating, and nausea. These symptoms can be due to the parasympathetic and sympathetic acute stress response to pain or to the effects of early cardiogenic shock. Of course, these same symptoms are caused by indigestion, chest wall muscle spasm, altitude adjustment, respiratory infection, and a host of other less serious problems. Where evacuation to medical care will be a high risk operation, we need to be able to decide if the complaint of chest pain indicates a serious problem. To help with this decision, we can evaluate the patient's risk factors for coronary artery disease.

Any patient with chest pain and a collection of risk factors should be considered at elevated risk for myocardial infarction and cardiac arrhythmia. Risk factors include disease states, genetics, medications, and lifestyle factors that contribute to narrowing and inflammation of the arteries supplying the heart. The more risk factors that your patient has, the more worried about his chest pain you should be.

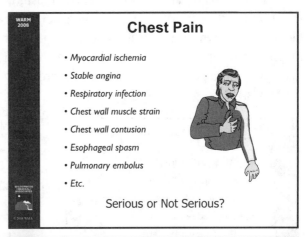

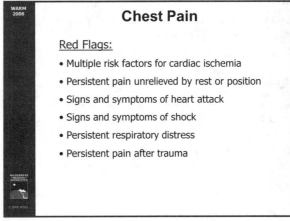

TREATMENT OF MYOCARDIAL ISCHEMIA

"Time is myocardium" is the mantra of treatment. The sooner the ischemia can be reversed, the less heart muscle will be damaged and the better the chance for survival. This means an urgent evacuation,

even if the patient cannot present to definitive medical care within the two-hour window for clot dissolving treatment.

The ideal evacuation would not increase the stress or level of exertion for your patient. But, you may find yourself choosing between a walk-out evacuation that takes an hour and a carry-out that may take several hours. You should favor the route that will put your patient under ALS care as soon as possible while causing the least increase in activity and myocardial oxygen demand.

As long as your patient is not already taking anticoagulant medications, give one adult aspirin tablet by mouth. This will reduce the tendency of the blood to clot, which may reduce ischemia in heart muscle. If the patient has other heart medication like nitroglycerin, assist him in taking it according to directions.

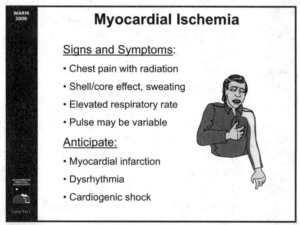

STABLE ANGINA

Your chest pain patient may give a history of stable angina: chest pain with exertion that resolves with rest. This develops when physical exertion increases the myocardial oxygen demand beyond the ability of chronically narrowed coronary arteries to supply it. The relative ischemia is temporary, assuming that the patient can reduce activity and oxygen demand.

If the pain does not resolve with rest, it may require that the patient use sub-lingual nitroglycerine tablets or spray. Nitroglycerine relaxes the smooth muscle of blood vessels to reduce the resistance to flow and thus the work the heart must do to circulate blood. Usually, a maximum of three doses of nitroglycerin is taken before referral to medical care is considered necessary. Pain that does not resolve as expected should be considered a heart attack and treated as such.

Patients with angina are at increased risk of myocardial infarction. Increased exertion and unexpected crisis in the backcountry can create a situation where rest is not possible. If persistent ischemia develops, definitive treatment is a long way off. This elevated level of risk should be discussed with any angina patient contemplating wilderness travel.

WARM 2008

Myocardial Ischemia

<u>Signs and Symptoms</u>:
- Chest pain with radiation
- Shell/core effect, sweating
- Elevated respiratory rate
- Pulse may be variable

<u>Anticipate</u>:
- Myocardial infarction
- Dysrhythmia
- Cardiogenic shock

WARM 2008

Myocardial Ischemia

<u>Specific Treatment</u>:
- Assist with nitroglycerin as prescribed
- Give one adult aspirin
- PROP
- Gentle but expeditious evacuation:
  - activity increases myocardial oxygen demand
  - time increases infarction
- ALS care as soon as possible

WARM 2008

Stable Angina

- History of chronic coronary artery constriction with *transient* myocardial ischemia
- Oxygen demand exceeds supply *temporarily*
- Exacerbated by exertion
- Relieved by rest
- Treated with nitroglycerin and oxygen
- May not represent an emergency

Diarrhea

29

One of the functions of the large intestine is to absorb fluid from feces just before excretion. This serves to conserve the body's fluid balance and allow you some degree of control over when and where excretion occurs. Diarrhea develops when the lining of the intestinal space is irritated by infection or toxins and fails to absorb fluid. The intestine can also leak more body fluid on its own, contributing to general fluid loss. Like abdominal pain, the generic assessment is serious or not serious. Diarrhea that is a softer version of normal stool and relatively infrequent in an otherwise healthy individual is usually not considered serious if fluid losses can be replaced by oral intake.

Diarrhea can be a symptom of other more serious problems, especially in the presence of abdominal pain. Diarrhea itself becomes a real problem when fluid loss occurs so rapidly that it cannot be replaced. For example, the cause of death in cholera is volume shock from dehydration due to diarrhea.

TREATMENT OF DIARRHEA

Mild diarrhea can be treated effectively with bismuth subsalicylate (Pepto-Bismol) or similar over-the-counter preparations. Narcotic antispasmodic drugs such as loprimide inhibit intestinal motility, allowing more time for the absorption of fluid. Beware of using loprimide if the cause of the diarrhea is bacterial infection, evidenced by blood or pus in the stool or the presence of fever. Obstructing drainage can increase the severity of the infection.

Replace fluid losses with oral or IV electrolyte solutions. Time will usually correct the situation, but if the problem persists longer than a week, medical advice should be sought. When red flag signs are noted, evacuation should be considered. If signs of volume shock are present, evacuation should be urgent if fluids cannot be replaced quickly in the field. During evacuation, oral fluids should be given as quickly as the patient can tolerate.

WARM 2008

Diarrhea

Red Flags:

- Associated with red flags for abdominal pain
- Fluid losses exceed intake
- Persistent fever
- Bloody diarrhea
- Signs of shock

WARM 2008

Diarrhea

Anticipate:

- Volume shock from dehydration

Treatment:

- Fluid and easily absorbed food
- Preserve body core temperature
- Loperamide (Imodium) if no red flags (4 mg x 1 dose, then 2 mg after each loose stool)
- Bismuth subsalicylate (Pepto-Bismol)
- Antibiotics for traveler's diarrhea

NOTES:

Constipation

30

The usual cause of constipation is dehydration. The large intestine absorbs fluid from feces producing a hard stool that is difficult to excrete. The patient reports fullness, cramping, and intermittent pain in the lower abdomen and pelvis.

Constipation becomes annoying when the patient feels bad because of it. Constipation becomes a problem when the rest of the body begins to suffer. Constipation becomes an emergency when associated with the red flags of abdominal pain. The less common but more serious causes include stool impaction, bowel obstruction, and neurologic deficit.

TREATMENT OF CONSTIPATION

Hydration is the best initial treatment and often relieves the problem. The next step is the use a stool softener and mild stimulant like the senna (Senokot) or docusate sodium (Colace). Mineral oil taken orally as an intestinal lubricant can reduce friction and allow stool to move. These treatments are very mild and generally very safe.

Laxatives like bisacodyl (Dulcolax) given orally or by suppository stimulate the bowel to contract. This is most effective and least painful after hydration and the administration of a stool softener. Laxatives can be dangerous if the patient has a bowel obstruction. Do not use these drugs in the presence of red flags for abdominal pain.

An enema is viewed by most people as the treatment of last resort. Warm water is instilled into the rectum by gravity feed. A small amount may be all that is necessary to lubricate and soften stool. An enema is also contraindicated with the red flags for abdominal pain.

Constipation can be prevented in the backcountry by staying well-hydrated and adding fiber to the diet. Carrying dehydrated or high-protein food can make this a challenge. Consider using a bulk agent like Metamucil Gel Caps to supplement your diet. It is also important to take the time and find the privacy for a decent bowel movement.

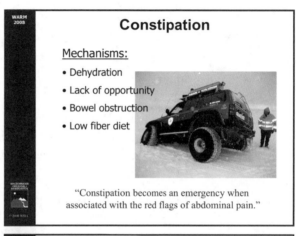

Constipation

WARM 2008

Mechanisms:

- Dehydration
- Lack of opportunity
- Bowel obstruction
- Low fiber diet

"Constipation becomes an emergency when associated with the red flags of abdominal pain."

Constipation

WARM 2008

Anticipate:

- Serious abdominal pain
- Systemic infection

Treatment:

- Hydration
- Stool softeners; Colace, Senokot
- Laxatives*; Dulcolax, Ex-lax
- Enema*

* Not in the presence of serious abdominal pain.

NOTES:

Nausea and Vomiting

31

Like diarrhea, vomiting can be the result of a problem with the gastrointestinal system or a symptom of other problems such as motion sickness, toxic ingestion, head injury, or infection. Finding and treating the primary cause is ideal. You must consider the additional problems that can be caused by severe fluid loss as well. Vomiting that is associated with the red flags for abdominal pain is considered serious.

TREATMENT OF VOMITING

Replacement of fluid loss is a priority. Because nausea inhibits oral intake, IV or rectal rehydration may be necessary. Oral intake may be successful if the patient can take small amounts frequently enough to maintain hydration. Look for normal urine output as evidence of success.

Airway obstruction and aspiration is an anticipated problem in any vomiting patient. Positioning for drainage and constant monitoring is important if the patient is not A on the AVPU scale or is exhibiting altered mental status. Keep somebody nearby to assist when necessary.

Antiemetic drugs can be given by intramuscular or intravenous injection orally, or by rectal suppository. The prescription drugs promethazine and compazine, and are examples. The over-the-counter antihistamines meclizine and diphenhydramine can be effective if the patient can tolerate oral medication. Acetaminophen is preferred over NSAIDs or oral narcotics for pain.

WARM 2008

Vomiting

Red Flags:
- Cannot control airway
- Cannot replace fluids
- Cannot maintain calories and body core temp
- Associated with red flags for abdominal pain

WARM 2008

Vomiting

Anticipate:
- Airway obstruction and aspiration
- Volume shock from dehydration

Treatment:
- Airway control
- Hydration and calories
- Maintain body core temperature
- Anti-emetic medication

NOTES:

Ear and Sinus Infection

32

EXTERNAL EAR INFECTION (SWIMMER'S EAR)

Swimmer's ear is a superficial bacterial infection of the external auditory canal. Also called external otitis, it develops when prolonged exposure to water leads to breakdown of the protective skin barrier. The signs and symptoms are not difficult to distinguish from middle ear infection.

Like any infection, it will be characterized by redness, warmth, swelling, and pain. The external structures of the ear and surrounding area will be tender to pressure and manipulation. The external ear canal may be swollen and obstructed.

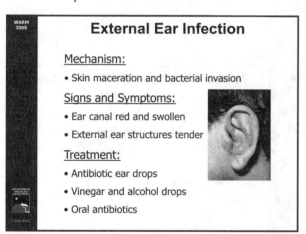

TREATMENT OF SWIMMERS EAR

Using mineral oil drops before swimming will reduce maceration of the skin and the incidence of infection. A few drops of vinegar combined with alcohol instilled into the ear canal after swimming is a good preventive treatment. There are also commercial preparations such as SwimEar™ available over the counter to help prevent external otitis. Do not use dry Q-tips because they will further irritate the ear canal.

Once the ear canal is infected, the ideal treatment is antibiotic eardrops, available in the United States only by prescription. Cortisporin® Otic Suspension is an example that combines the antibiotic neosporin with the topical steroid cortisone.

MIDDLE EAR INFECTION AND SINUSITIS

The sinus cavity referred to as the *middle ear* lies behind the ear drum and extends through a narrow opening into the nasopharynx. Like the other sinus cavities inside the skull, the middle ear is lined with mucous membrane and drained through one small opening. In the healthy individual, mucous is continuously produced and drained through the eustachian tube into the throat where it is swallowed. Problems begin when the tube becomes obstructed by swelling and inflammation from a viral infection or as the result of irritation by seawater or smoke. The trapped mucous provides a growth medium for bacteria, and a middle ear infection develops.

The typical symptom of middle ear infection is pain. Bending over at the waist increases pressure in the affected ear and increases the pain. Middle ear infection can be differentiated from swimmer's ear by the fact that, although the ear hurts, the external

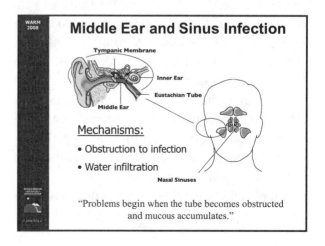

ear structures and ear canal are not red, swollen, or tender to touch.

The problem called *sinusitis* develops by the same mechanism in the frontal, maxillary, or ethmoid sinuses in the skull. Typical symptoms include pain, pressure, and sometimes a green or bloody nasal discharge. An infection in the maxillary sinus in the face can act like dental infection in the upper teeth, but you won't find a specific tooth that is tender to percussion.

Red flags for middle ear and sinus infection reflect the anticipated problem of spread to adjacent structures like the skull, inner ear, and brain. Persistent fever, severe pain, or obvious swelling in the face or neck indicates a potentially serious condition and warrants emergency evacuation and early access to antibiotics. Any change in mental status or the development of persistent vomiting could indicate involvement of the brain.

TREATMENT OF MIDDLE EAR INFECTION AND SINUSITIS

As with any obstructed organ, the situation can be improved with drainage. Try to reduce the swelling and obstruction of the eustachian tube and sinus passages with decongestant nasal spray or by having the patient breath steam from a pot of hot water. Keeping your patient well hydrated is important. This will keep mucous from drying and becoming too thick to drain.

Antibiotics are sometimes necessary for complete treatment of middle ear and sinus infections and are recommended if the patient is not responding to decongestion and hydration. A middle ear infection may ultimately perforate the eardrum and drain spontaneously through the external ear canal. Pain is almost immediately relieved as the pressure is released, but hearing may be temporarily impaired. If no fever or other adverse symptoms develop, there is no emergency. Avoid swimming and diving, and see a medical practitioner when possible.

Treating infection of the other sinus cavities is similar, except that there is no safety valve like the eardrum through which they can perforate and drain if necessary. Aggressive decongestion and hydration is necessary to promote drainage through the sinus passages. Sinus infection not responding to field treatment is best evacuated to medical care, especially if moderate pain or fever is present. Steroid nasal sprays may be prescribed to reduce inflammation and swelling. Antibiotic therapy, sometimes for several weeks, is indicated in resistant cases.

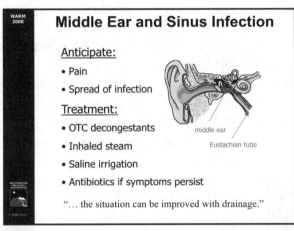

Middle Ear and Sinus Infection

Anticipate:
- Pain
- Spread of infection

Treatment:
- OTC decongestants
- Inhaled steam
- Saline irrigation
- Antibiotics if symptoms persist

"… the situation can be improved with drainage."

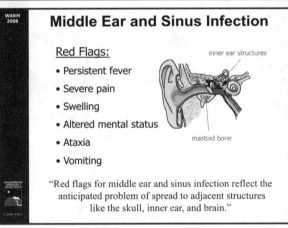

Middle Ear and Sinus Infection

Red Flags:
- Persistent fever
- Severe pain
- Swelling
- Altered mental status
- Ataxia
- Vomiting

"Red flags for middle ear and sinus infection reflect the anticipated problem of spread to adjacent structures like the skull, inner ear, and brain."

Nosebleed

33

Most nosebleeds occur in an area of the anterior nostril called *Kesselbach's Plexus*. Bleeding from here will drain out of the nose if the patient is positioned upright with the head forward. When the bleed starts spontaneously or as a result of nose picking, the problem is generally uncomplicated. Bleeding will stop quickly with direct pressure. However, if the bleeding is the result of facial trauma, you should consider the possibility of facial bone fracture.

In rare cases bleeding can originate in the posterior nasopharynx. Applying direct pressure can be impossible. If a patient is using anti-coagulant medications or even a lot of aspirin, bleeding can be significant.

TREATMENT OF NOSEBLEED

Position the patient sitting forward or lying face down to allow for drainage out of the nose rather than down the throat. Instruct her to blow out any clots, then pinch the nostrils together and hold firmly *for 15 minutes*. This applies simple direct pressure to the most likely bleeding source. Like any bleeding, it is essential to hold enough pressure for a long enough time. This will stop most nosebleeds that you are likely to see.

Persistent bleeds can be treated with nasal packing. A light-flow (small size) tampon can be gently inserted into the nostril for several hours. Soaking the tampon with a few drops of a decongestant nasal spray like oxymetazalone (the vasoconstrictor in Afrin®) will reduce bleeding by constricting blood vessels in the nasal mucosa. The packing should be removed within four hours or so. The frequency of nose bleeds from dry air and high altitude can be reduced by coating the inside of the nostril with Vaseline or antibiotic ointment periodically. New powdered clot-enhancers are now available over the counter for nuisance bleeding, including nosebleeds.

As with any other bleeding, nosebleed becomes serious when volume shock is anticipated. If you cannot control a severe nosebleed in the field, make the patient as comfortable as possible and prepare for an urgent evacuation. If the patient needs to lie down, protect the airway by positioning her face down or on her side with the chest and head supported to allow for drainage from the nose and mouth. A carry-out evacuation may be necessary if volume shock develops.

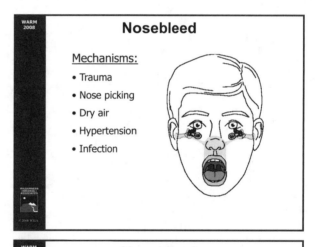

WARM 2008

Nosebleed

Mechanisms:
- Trauma
- Nose picking
- Dry air
- Hypertension
- Infection

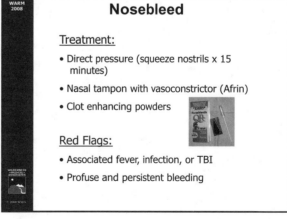

WARM 2008

Nosebleed

Treatment:
- Direct pressure (squeeze nostrils x 15 minutes)
- Nasal tampon with vasoconstrictor (Afrin)
- Clot enhancing powders

Red Flags:
- Associated fever, infection, or TBI
- Profuse and persistent bleeding

NOTES:

Urinary Tract Infection

34

Uncomplicated and easily treated urinary tract infections (UTIs) are generally limited to women. Because the female urethra is only a few centimeters long, it is fairly easy for normal skin or intestinal bacteria to migrate from the outside into the bladder. Normal urination flushes bacteria out of the urethra, preventing this from happening, but this system can be upset in a number of ways.

Perhaps the most common cause in wilderness travelers is urinary retention. This is usually due to dehydration or simply through lack of opportunity to urinate. Getting out of a warm sleeping bag, bracing yourself against the pitch and roll of a small boat at sea, or negotiating relief around a climbing harness on a big wall can inhibit frequent flushing. Any bacteria entering the bladder and urethra have a longer period of time in which to multiply and invade the mucosal lining.

Another predisposing factor for urinary tract infection is inadequate hygiene. In settings where bathing is difficult the number of bacteria on the outer surface of the skin increases dramatically and makes infection more likely.

A third factor is direct trauma to the urethra. The usual culprit is frequent or vigorous sexual activity, but inflammation can also be caused by horseback riding, biking, or a tight wetsuit. The urethral opening becomes inflamed, is invaded by bacteria, and infection results.

More complicated and dangerous infections can develop when the bacteria climb beyond the bladder to invade the ureters and kidney. Sexually transmitted diseases are also considered more dangerous because the bacteria or virus is foreign to the body and is more difficult to eradicate. In the male where the urethra is much longer, acute infection of the urinary tract is unusual and may indicate a complicated condition. The most common cause is sexually transmitted disease.

The signs and symptoms of uncomplicated urinary tract infection include low pelvic pain, frequent urination in small amounts, cloudy urine, and pain, tingling, or burning on urination. It is possible to confuse uncomplicated urinary tract infection with a vaginal infection because the inflamed vaginal mucosa and external genitalia may sting and itch on contact with urine.

TREATMENT OF URINARY TRACT INFECTION

Cranberry juice or cranberry tablets can sometimes

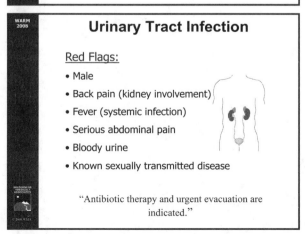

WARM 2008

Urinary Tract Infection

Mechanisms:
- Obstruction
- Dehydration
- Inadequate hygiene
- Localized trauma.

Treatment:
- Hydration
- Antibiotics

WARM 2008

Urinary Tract Infection

Red Flags:
- Male
- Back pain (kidney involvement)
- Fever (systemic infection)
- Serious abdominal pain
- Bloody urine
- Known sexually transmitted disease

"Antibiotic therapy and urgent evacuation are indicated."

help prevent infection, but the standard of care for uncomplicated urinary tract infection is oral antibiotics. Treatment regimens can be as short as one dose, but three to seven days is more typical and effective. Temporary measures, pending access to medical care, involve treating UTI with drainage and cleansing like any other soft tissue infection. Keep the external genitalia as clean as possible and drink plenty of fluids to promote frequent urination.

Signs and symptoms that indicate that infection has progressed beyond the superficial lining of the urethra and bladder indicate a more serious condition. These include fever, back pain, and blood in the urine. The possibility of sexually transmitted disease should also be considered a red flag. Antibiotic therapy and urgent evacuation are indicated.

NOTES:

Vaginitis

35

Infection of the vagina occurs when something upsets the normal balance between yeast and bacteria allowing one of the species to grow out of control. Antibiotics taken for a strep throat, for example, will kill many of the bacteria in the vagina, allowing for an overgrowth of yeast. Changes in the vaginal environment can also be caused by clothing, sexual activity, stress, dehydration, and other factors.

Yeast infection is more common than bacterial. Signs and symptoms include itching or burning, and a whitish or "cheesy" vaginal discharge. There may also be tingling or burning as urine irritates inflamed tissues, causing some confusion with urinary tract infection. The practitioner will need to ask specific questions about the presence of discharge and the location of discomfort to make the distinction.

Many women presenting with yeast vaginitis will have a previous history of similar symptoms and will recognize the problem and know the treatment. New onset cases with no previous history should be taken more seriously. Even if an uncomplicated yeast infection is suspected, medical evaluation is indicated.

Bacterial vaginitis also causes itching and burning, but the discharge is typically yellow or brown and malodorous. A lost tampon is a common cause.

Medication use, diabetes, and other systemic problems can also contribute.

Vaginitis becomes an emergency when it migrates into the uterus and fallopian tubes causing the infection known as pelvic inflammatory disease. The symptoms will include the easily recognized red flags for abdominal pain. Sexually transmitted disease should also be considered a red flag.

TREATMENT OF VAGINITIS

Simple yeast vaginitis may respond to non-prescription treatment in the field. Medications like miconazole (Monistat) suppositories are available over the counter and should be carried on expedition. The manufacturers warn against relying on this treatment unless the patient is fairly certain of the diagnosis through past experience.

Because yeast and bacteria grow well in a warm and moist environment, the situation can also be improved by staying dry and cool. This means wearing loose fitting clothing and spending less time in the wet suit. Frequent bathing is also important.

Bacterial vaginitis is best evaluated and treated in a medical facility. Practitioners will want to rule out sexually transmitted disease and treat with antibiotics. Evacuation need not be an emergency if symptoms are not progressing and no fever or pain is noted.

When evacuation or definitive treatment is not available, a reduction of symptoms or complete field cure may be achieved by using a douche of dilute povidone iodine or vinegar and water. Add a tablespoon of povidone iodine solution or vinegar to a quart of water and instruct your patient to douche once a day for several days. This will be most effective when your patient can spend several hours supine after treatment.

Douching is not a high-tech operation. It can be

WARM 2008

Vaginitis

Treatment:
- Yeast Infection:
  - fluconazole tablet (Diflucan, Rx)
  - topical antifungal (Monistat)
  - 1% PI douche x 3 days
- Bacterial Vaginitis:
  - oral or vaginal antibiotics
  - 1% PI douche x 3 days
  - evacuation for medical evaluation

WILDERNESS MEDICAL ASSOCIATES

© 2008 WMA

accomplished using a regular hydration system or 60 cc catheter tip syringe and nasopharyngeal airway. Anything similar will work, but fluid should not be forced into the vagina under pressure. Gravity feed is sufficient. A douche should not be used by a pregnant patient or if trauma is suspected.

NOTES:

Testicular Pain

36

Like any other organ, testicles can become obstructed, infected, or ischemic. A rare but dangerous cause of sudden onset pain is testicular torsion, where the testicle twists inside the scrotum impinging its blood supply. Ischemia causes pain and will result in infarction of the testicle if not corrected. Testicular torsion can sometimes be relieved by gently elevating the scrotum and allowing the testicle to spontaneously unwind. Even if this maneuver is successful and pain is relieved, non-emergent medical follow up is advised. Persistent pain unrelieved by this procedure should be considered an emergency. Persistent pain following trauma is also of concern, especially if swelling is severe. Immediate evacuation to surgical care is indicated.

Infection of the testes or epididymis is more common than torsion, but still unusual. It is extremely uncomfortable and potentially serious. Persistent testicular pain with or without swelling should motivate an emergency evacuation. Antibiotics can be used if evacuation is delayed or impossible. Epididymitis can be difficult to distinguish from testicular torsion.

NOTES:

Respiratory Infection

37

Like abdominal pain, respiratory infections have a variety of causes and effects. Pneumonia is an infection of lung tissue, resulting in the accumulation of pus or serous exudate in the alveoli. Bronchitis is an infection of the bronchial tubes of the lower airway causing lower airway constriction. Pharyngitis, tonsillitis, and epiglottitis are infections of the structures in the upper airway. Pleurisy involves the chest wall and outer surface of the lung.

In the field it can be difficult to tell one from another. The diagnosis often remains generic: serious or not serious? Is this infection respiratory distress?

The vast majority of mild respiratory infections that we call a *cold* or *flu* are caused by viruses. They typically produce a constellation of symptoms such as runny nose, mild headache, sneezing, coughing, irritated eyes, mild sore throat, muscular aches, and intermittent fever. The patient is usually not impaired in his ability to perform normal tasks and continues to eat, drink, urinate, and produce stool more or less on schedule. Respiratory distress is not significant.

Problems develop when the virus is particularly virulent or the viral infection opens the way for a secondary bacterial infection. This is how patients who start with a cold can end up with a bacterial pneumonia, bronchitis, or strep throat. More serious

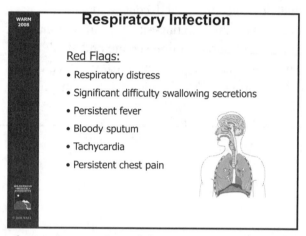

Respiratory Infection

Red Flags:
- Respiratory distress
- Significant difficulty swallowing secretions
- Persistent fever
- Bloody sputum
- Tachycardia
- Persistent chest pain

infections are indicated by a cough productive of thick yellow, green, or brown sputum. The patient may experience chills, shortness of breath, and chest pain on respiration. You may hear wheezing, or fine or coarse crackles when listening to the chest with your stethoscope. Fever will be more persistent. Respiratory infection becomes an emergency when it causes respiratory distress or interferes significantly with eating and drinking.

TREATMENT OF RESPIRATORY INFECTION

Although anti-viral drugs may be effective in the early stages of a cold or flu, eradication of the virus

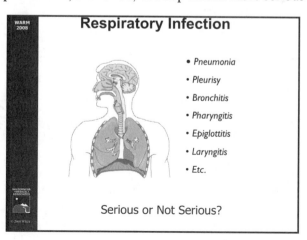

Respiratory Infection

- *Pneumonia*
- *Pleurisy*
- *Bronchitis*
- *Pharyngitis*
- *Epiglottitis*
- *Laryngitis*
- *Etc.*

Serious or Not Serious?

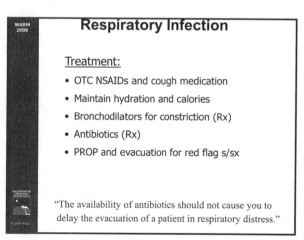

Respiratory Infection

Treatment:
- OTC NSAIDs and cough medication
- Maintain hydration and calories
- Bronchodilators for constriction (Rx)
- Antibiotics (Rx)
- PROP and evacuation for red flag s/sx

"The availability of antibiotics should not cause you to delay the evacuation of a patient in respiratory distress."

will usually depend on the body's immune system. The patient with the constellation of mild symptoms suggestive of viral infection should be made more comfortable while the body works to defeat the virus. Use whatever over-the-counter medications make the patient feel better while not interfering with his ability to function. Local decongestants such as nasal sprays, systemic decongestants, and non-narcotic cough medications can be very helpful at alleviating symptoms, as do anti-inflammatory medications like ibuprofen. Equally important is maintaining fluid balance, eating well, staying warm, and getting enough rest. This reduces the number of stressors that the body has to deal with.

The patient with symptoms of bacterial infection may need antibiotics, especially if wheezing, rales, or rhonchi are detected on auscultation of the lungs. If you are authorized to use these drugs, the patient can safely be treated in the field if he is doing well otherwise. The availability of antibiotics should not cause you to delay the evacuation of a patient in respiratory distress.

NOTES:

Sore Throat

38

Most sore throats are caused by viral infection and occur as part of a constellation of symptoms related to a cold or flu. These are self-limiting and require only symptomatic treatment. However, you must monitor for the development of severe infection where swelling of the tonsils, epiglottis, and uvula have the potential to cause airway obstruction.

This will most often be the result of a bacterial infection such as strep throat or epiglotitis, but it can occur with viral mononucleosis. Bacterial infection is characterized by persistent pain, difficulty swallowing, and obvious edema of pharyngeal structures. Pus can be seen as white patches on the throat and tonsils. Fever tends to be persistent. Suspected bacterial infection should be seen by a medical practitioner. Mild pharyngitis can be effectively treated with ibuprofen, cool liquids, and topical medication like throat lozenges.

Impending airway obstruction is suggested by the patient's inability to swallow secretions or water. He may position himself in a chin-thrust to keep the airway open. Stridor may be noted. This is a medical emergency in which evacuation and advanced life support is indicated. In a desperate situation, epinephrine may be used by advanced providers to temporarily reduce swelling and keep the airway open. Steroids like prednisone may also help, but will take several hours to have any effect.

NOTES:

Dental Trauma and Infection

39

DENTAL TRAUMA

Loose teeth, tooth fragments, blood, and swollen tissues can result in airway obstruction. The mechanism of injury can be associated with brain and spine injury. Pain can produce ASR. Swallowing blood can cause vomiting. The initial assessment of dental trauma is directed at ensuring that critical body system problems are considered and stabilized. Beyond that, broken teeth do not represent a medical emergency.

TREATMENT OF DENTAL TRAUMA

Position the patient to allow drainage of blood and debris out of the mouth, rather than down the throat. Instruct the patient to rinse the mouth with cool water. This will clean out blood clots and loose teeth and help to stop bleeding. Examine the mouth with a good light. Look for teeth that are loose or fractured but still in the socket. Look for empty sockets that could match any avulsed teeth you may have found.

Teeth that have been cleanly avulsed have a fair chance of reattaching if returned to their socket within a few hours. Handle the tooth only by the enamel, not by its root. Rinse the tooth in clean water and push

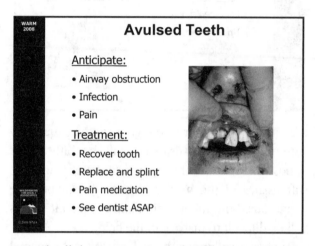

Avulsed Teeth

Anticipate:
- Airway obstruction
- Infection
- Pain

Treatment:
- Recover tooth
- Replace and splint
- Pain medication
- See dentist ASAP

it gently all the way into its socket. You can splint the tooth to a healthy one adjacent to it by tying it with dental floss or fishing line or by constructing a bridge from dental wax or Cavit. Any teeth that are loose, but still in the socket, may be splinted in this manner as well.

Fractured teeth that are still in place may be extremely sensitive on exposure to air if the nerve is still alive. The fracture site can be anesthetized and disinfected with topical oral pain relievers like oil of cloves and covered with temporary filling material or dental wax. The loss of a filling can be treated the same way using wax or filling material to protect the sensitive nerve tissue that is exposed when the filling falls out. Loose fillings or crowns can also be temporarily glued back in place with toothpaste. The patient should eat only soft foods and cool liquids.

Referral of trauma or lost fillings to dental follow-up may be non-emergent if infection does not develop. In significant trauma where teeth have been avulsed or fractured, prophylactic antibiotics are indicated. Pain medication and a soft diet may also be required.

DENTAL INFECTION

Infection and swelling within the confined space at

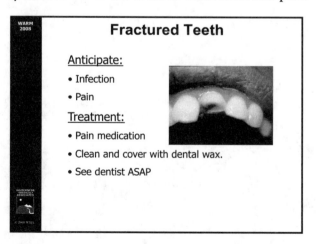

Fractured Teeth

Anticipate:
- Infection
- Pain

Treatment:
- Pain medication
- Clean and cover with dental wax.
- See dentist ASAP

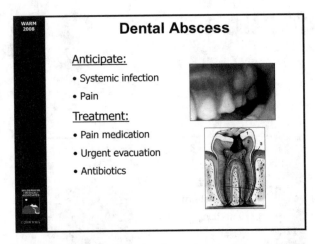

WARM
2008

Dental Abscess

Anticipate:

• Systemic infection

• Pain

Treatment:

• Pain medication

• Urgent evacuation

• Antibiotics

the base of a tooth or in the gum can be exquisitely painful. Eating and drinking will be difficult or impossible. If the infection penetrates into the soft tissues of the head and neck, it can become dangerous. Both the infection and the pain it causes will be difficult to manage in the field.

Bacteria usually enter through a break in the enamel caused by trauma or a cavity and form an abscess with the typical swelling, pressure, and pain. Swelling of the gum on the effected side may be evident, as well as the tenderness of one or more teeth when tapped with a finger or stick. A patient with a more serious infection will show facial swelling and fever.

TREATMENT OF DENTAL INFECTION

The treatment of a dental infection includes drainage, antibiotics, and pain relief. The preferred method is drilling and cleaning the inside of the tooth and installing a filling. Antibiotics are used to bring the infection under control, and pain relievers are usually necessary. Urgent evacuation to dental care is indicated if swelling, fever, or severe pain is present.

Temporary pain relief may be obtained with topical pain relievers like Orabase or oil of cloves, and oral or injectable pain medication. If immediate evacuation is not possible, begin high-dose antibiotics and warm compresses. This may reduce the severity of the infection pending evacuation to dental care. In a worst-case scenario, remember that up until quite recently in dental history pulling the tooth was the definitive treatment for dental infection.

NOTES:

Eye Problems

40

The common terms *red eye*, *pink eye*, or *conjunctivitis* refer to inflammation of the thin membranous lining of the eye and the inside of the eye lids (conjunctiva). There are a number of causes, including infection, sunburn, foreign body, trauma, chemical irritation, or even fatigue. It can also represent one of the symptoms of a more serious condition like glaucoma.

All the various causes of conjunctivitis produce similar symptoms. The patient will complain of an itching or burning sensation, tearing, and photophobia. The eye will appear red as conjunctival blood vessels dilate in response to inflammation. There may be a small amount of eyelid swelling.

In uncomplicated cases, the cornea will remain clear, the pupil will continue to react to light, and vision will be unaffected except for transient blurring caused by tears or exudate. Normal eye movements, called *extraocular movements*, might be uncomfortable, but fully intact. There will be no evidence of blood inside the eye, and the patient will not complain of a headache.

Red flags indicating a more severe case include clouding of the cornea, persistent visual disturbances, or severe headache. The examiner may note bleeding inside the eye, appearing as a red or brown

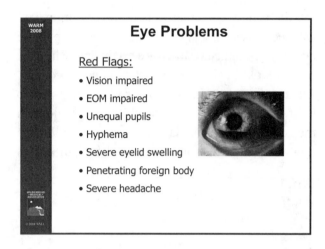

Eye Problems

Red Flags:
- Vision impaired
- EOM impaired
- Unequal pupils
- Hyphema
- Severe eyelid swelling
- Penetrating foreign body
- Severe headache

discoloration behind the lower portion of the cornea (hyphema). Extraocular movements may be inhibited or very painful. The pupils may not react equally to light. Lid swelling may be severe. These signs and symptoms should prompt early evacuation.

TREATMENT OF CONJUNCTIVITIS

The generic treatment for conjunctival irritation includes systemic pain medications, lubricating eye drops, and protective lenses. Antibiotic eye drops or ointment is applied when infection is present. An eye patch is used only when extraoccular movements will cause further harm, such as with an imbedded or penetrating foreign body.

An ophthalmic anesthetic, such as Tetracaine, is often used by clinicians during eye examinations and foreign body removal. One or two drops will numb the conjunctiva and cornea for up to an hour. These anesthetics should not be used for routine pain relief or treatment. It could mask the development of a severe condition or allow the patient to cause further injury without realizing it.

Sand or other debris that gets onto the conjunctiva will cause immediate irritation, redness, and tearing.

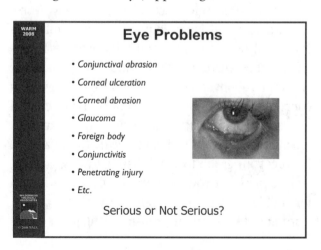

Eye Problems

- *Conjunctival abrasion*
- *Corneal ulceration*
- *Corneal abrasion*
- *Glaucoma*
- *Foreign body*
- *Conjunctivitis*
- *Penetrating injury*
- *Etc.*

Serious or Not Serious?

Onset is usually abrupt, and the cause often obvious. The easiest and least traumatic way to remove something from the eye is by irrigation with water. The simplest methods are to have the patient immerse his face in clean water and blink his eyes or to irrigate with your water bottle.

If the patient continues to have the sensation, you will need to examine the conjunctiva. Gently pull the lids away from the eye and use a bright light while the patient looks in all directions. If you find something, use a wet cotton swab or corner of a gauze pad to lift it off the membrane. If the object is imbedded in the conjunctiva or cornea and resists your efforts to remove it, leave it alone. Imbedded foreign bodies

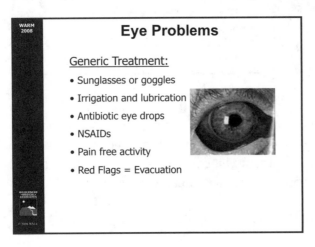

Eye Problems

Generic Treatment:

- Sunglasses or goggles
- Irrigation and lubrication
- Antibiotic eye drops
- NSAIDs
- Pain free activity
- Red Flags = Evacuation

require medical attention. Patch the eye if safe to do so, and plan to walk out. Beware of using a patch in situations where impaired vision could be dangerous.

The cornea is structurally tough but neurologically sensitive. Its outer surface can be scratched by a foreign body, branch, fingernail, or wind-blown ice crystals. Corneal abrasion can cause considerable pain and inflammation, making the patient feel like something is in the eye. Sometimes the abrasion can be seen by shining a flashlight across the eye from the side. Corneal abrasions are usually more annoying than serious. As long as no red flags are present, treatment may be generic and symptomatic. Healing usually occurs within 72 hours.

Ultraviolet light can burn the conjunctiva and cornea just as it does unprotected skin. The result is the same: pain, redness, and swelling. The examination will reveal that the inflammation is limited to the sun-exposed part of the eye, leaving the conjunctiva under the lids unaffected. In severe cases, the cornea may become pitted and cloudy in appearance, causing the condition known as *snow blindness*. Fortunately UV rays do not penetrate deeply, so damage is usually superficial. Symptomatic treatment with lubricating drops, pain medication, and protective lenses will allow healing over several days.

A viral or bacterial infection of the conjunctiva is what most people mean by the term *conjunctivitis* or pink eye. The typical signs and symptoms include a yellow or green discharge that can stick the eyelids together during sleep. The eyelids themselves may appear slightly puffy and reddened. The conjunctiva will appear red with inflammation. The patient will complain of an itching or burning sensation that may resemble a foreign body.

A mild superficial infection will not cause a headache or severe lid edema. Vision will be blurred when tears or pus pass over the pupil, but otherwise unaffected. Pain will be annoying but not severe. The cornea remains clear, pupils respond normally to light, and extraocular movements are intact.

Most mild bacterial and viral conjunctivitis will resolve spontaneously, but this is difficult to predict. You should allow the eyes to drain. Do not use a patch. Field treatment using frequent irrigation and warm soaks may improve the symptoms.

Treatment with antibiotics, either orally or as eye drops, is the preferred treatment, especially if symptoms appear to become progressively worse rather than stabilizing or improving. Severe infection evidenced by severe pain and lid swelling warrants an urgent evacuation. You should be particularly concerned about conjunctivitis in the patient wearing contact lenses. The lenses should be removed and not reused. Special antibiotics may be necessary.

Note that an eye infection can be quite contagious. Instruct your group to avoid sharing towels, goggles, or face masks. If you have access and authorization for antibiotic drops or ointment, treat both eyes.

Irritants like soap and caustic plant juices cause

chemical conjunctivitis. In mild cases, the cornea remains clear. In severe cases, it may be pitted or cloudy in appearance. The treatment for chemical exposure is copious irrigation with water or saline solution. Expect mild redness following prolonged irrigation, but it should begin to resolve within several hours following treatment. If it gets worse, the chemical may still be present. Irrigation should be repeated and evacuation considered.

Contact lenses are another frequent cause of inflammation, especially at altitude. Dry air and reduced oxygen availability can cause corneal damage. Affected patients should use lubricating eye drops and allow their eyes as many lens-free hours per day as possible.

NOTES:

Section VI
Roles and Responsibilities
of the Medical Practitioner

Expedition Medicine and Experiental Education

41

The informal title "doc" is given to an army platoon's medic, regardless of the level of the medic's training and certification. It recognizes the medic's special role as lifesaver, caregiver, and confidant to the soldiers that he or she is assigned to. Whether in combat, civilian SAR operations, or on a sailing expedition, the role of the medical officer is unique and demanding. In some circumstances, the task can be considerably more complex and challenging than that filled by an emergency physician in a hospital.

In most situations, you become an educator and safety officer as well as a medical practitioner. It may be your job to brief your traveling companions on safety concerns, environmental threats, and preexisting conditions among those in your group. Also, by default or design, you may be the only one anticipating and planning for rescue and evacuation. The more you can anticipate and address problems before a crisis develops, the more time you will have to deal with the unexpected issues that inevitably arise.

You will need a working knowledge of local environmental conditions, medical resources, and the condition of your crew. You should also be intimately familiar with the equipment and medication that you carry. Your confidence and competence will be

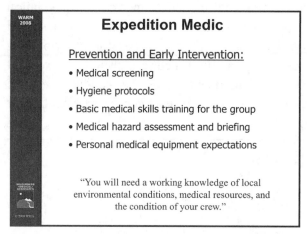

directly related to the quality of your preparation. Finally, the scope of your role and responsibilities, as well as your limitations, should be clearly understood by all concerned.

Pre-trip screening discussions with clients and their medical advisors has also become a normal and expected part of the job. Recent trends in adventure travel and experiential education now require a greater understanding of chronic disease states and the ability to make reasonable risk/benefit decisions with your clients. People with angina, asthma, and diabetes are as interested in trekking and sailing as anyone else, and it is no longer routine practice to exclude them.

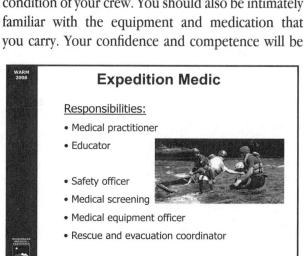

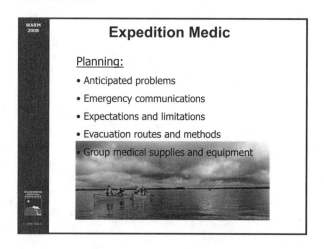

If you will be serving as the expedition medic or instructor who will responsible for a client with a chronic condition, it may be appropriate (with the patient's permission) for you to have a direct discussion with her normal medical practioner. Between your expertise in backcountry travel and wilderness medicine and the medical person's clinical experience and knowledge of the patient, you should be able to assess the risk involved in the trip being contemplated. The patient can also be an excellent source of information about her condition and the proper response to emergencies. Diabetics, for example, are usually very well informed about their disease and can help to further *your* understanding of the condition.

In the end though, the decision to accept responsibility for the care of a client with a preexisting and potentially dangerous medical condition should be yours. If the anticipated problem becomes real, you and your group will be the ones dealing with it. It is not practical or reasonable to defer this judgment solely to a physician who will not be traveling with you and who may not fully understand the environmental and logistical challenges.

NOTES:

The Medical Role in Search and Rescue

42

In a large-scale disaster response or SAR operations, there will be a number of medical roles to fill from field treatment to medical control. By contrast, a small team on a limited mission may field only one medical officer. Whatever the situation, and for any role to which you are assigned, you should know who you are working for, who is working for you, what you are doing, and how long you are expected to do it. Knowing something about the *Incident Command System (ICS)* will help.

The ICS is used in one form or another in most fire, rescue, and disaster situations. The depth and complexity will vary with the size and duration of the mission. The Incident Commander (IC) has

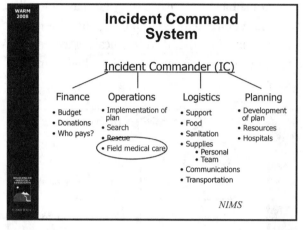

responsibility for the entire operation. Supervision of field operations, where most medical personnel are deployed, is usually delegated to an Operations Section Chief, usually stationed at or near the incident site. This section chief directs *Branch, Division,* or *Group Leaders* responsible for specific tasks or geographic areas.

ICS and SAR management is beyond the scope of this text. But, if you choose to become involved in search and rescue it is certainly wise to become familiar with the system and how it might be used by any team with which you will deploy, and to know where you fit in as a medical provider. If you are responding to an unfamiliar operation, look for the

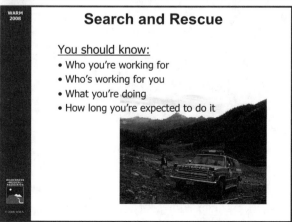

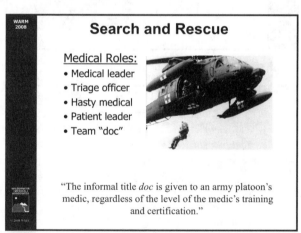

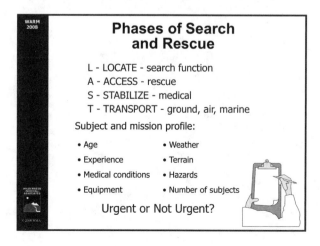

IC or command post (CP). In the field, look for the operations section chief or medical leader.

How you prepare your response will be determined by the type of incident. A known medical problem at a known location allows you to be fairly specific in your choice of equipment and personnel. A search for a lost subject who may or may not have a medical problem requires a totally different plan. This is basic information that the field medical officer should obtain in a briefing from the section chief or medical leader.

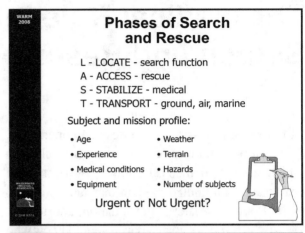

Phases of Search and Rescue

L - LOCATE - search function
A - ACCESS - rescue
S - STABILIZE - medical
T - TRANSPORT - ground, air, marine

Subject and mission profile:

- Age
- Experience
- Medical conditions
- Equipment
- Weather
- Terrain
- Hazards
- Number of subjects

Urgent or Not Urgent?

Type of Response

Known Location	Known Location
Known Medical	Unknown Medical
Known Medical	Unknown Location
Unknown Location	Unknown Medical

"How you prepare your response will be determined by the type of incident."

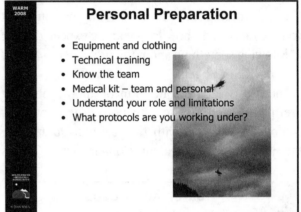

Personal Preparation

- Equipment and clothing
- Technical training
- Know the team
- Medical kit – team and personal
- Understand your role and limitations
- What protocols are you working under?

NOTES:

Section VII

Organization, Equipment and Materials

Appropriate Technology for Wilderness and Rescue Medicine

43

The size and weight of medical supplies and equipment carried will be determined by how you transport it, the role you fill, your level of training, and the number of people to be covered. Boats, rafts, and trucks are certainly less limiting than the need to fit everything in a belt pack. Mariners and motorized rescuers can usually find space for dedicated splinting materials, irrigation solutions, and other bulky supplies. The practitioner who backpacks a medical kit will need to be much more discriminating.

Some of the equipment and material used in the emergency department will function well in the backcountry, most will not. Appropriate medical technology for the offshore and wilderness environment is closer to that used by veterinarians and home health care nurses. You are looking for equipment that is simple and light with few moving parts. Bandages and dressings will need to survive harsh conditions but be simple to apply. Medications should not require close monitoring, prolonged administration, or cause unacceptable side effects.

A simple pocket mask or White Pulmonary Resuscitator connected to a helpful rescuer will provide heated and humidified ventilations without the weight and complexity of an oxygen-powered system with an external heat source. Vet wrap, an elastic bandage originally designed for livestock, will stand up to mud and rain much better than the white roller gauze found in the emergency department. Pain medication that can be administered by mouth, rectum, or intramuscular injection will be easier to manage than anything that requires an intravenous line.

Carrying traction or long leg splints for the lower extremity is generally not necessary. A well-padded litter effectively splints everything from the neck through the tibia. Stabilization of ankle, wrist, hands, and forearm injuries can be accomplished with a simple SAM® splint or any rigid object. Add a sling and you can include the elbow, upper arm, and clavicle.

Oxygen is administered for almost everything on the ambulance, but in the wilderness setting we look for a good reason to carry this relatively heavy and bulky equipment. You might choose to leave it behind when responding to an unknown problem at an unknown location. But, oxygen is certainly worth packing when responding to a known or suspected critical system problem at a known location.

The AED falls into the same category. You may choose to carry the device, along with the oxygen and cardiac medications, when responding to a known cardiac problem. Otherwise, the likelihood of use does not justify its weight and bulk in your pack.

On most trips, it makes sense to arrange your kit in modules. Put the materials used for minor maintenance and repair like Band-Aids and antibiotic ointment in a separate container. This module will have as much to do with preventing medical problems as treating them, and it should be easily accessible. It may work best for each member of the team to have their own. The more critical but less frequently used supplies can be kept elsewhere.

MEDICATIONS

Medications should be repackaged to prevent damage from moisture and movement. A bottle of loose pills will turn into powder after a few hours on the trail. Pack the contents tight with cotton or gauze in a waterproof vial, and add a few grains of dry rice to absorb any stray moisture. Any prescription medications should be accompanied by documentation from the prescribing practitioner, especially if you will be crossing international borders. Include written instructions for the use of the medication. For each medication, you should know:

Actions: How the drug works. Epinephrine, for example, constricts blood vessels and dilates bronchial tubes. Ibuprofen inhibits the chemical mediators of pain and inflammation.

Indications: What the drug is for. For our purposes, epinephrine is used to treat asthma and anaphylaxis. Ibuprofen reduces pain, inflammation, and fever.

Contraindications: When the drug should not be used. Ibuprofen, for example, should not be used when there is a potential for life-threatening bleeding because it reduces blood clotting.

Side Effects: Secondary effects of the drug that may or may not be desirable or acceptable. For example, drowsiness is a side effect of diphenhydramine. This may be useful or dangerous, depending on the situation. Allergies are an undesirable side effect that can occur with any medication.

Dosage and Route: How much is given how often? Is it by mouth, by injection, absorbed by the mucous membranes of the nose or mouth, absorbed through the skin, or given rectally.

FLUID

Fluid resuscitation is desirable for the patient in shock from dehydration. The ideal treatment is IV fluid replacement, but this is not always practical. Oral fluid replacement with electrolyte solutions can be very effective if the patient can swallow safely and is not vomiting. Rectal fluid replacement is another option, but more difficult to manage and somewhat slower. In many cases where dehydration is the primary mechanism, field rehydration can make a carry-out evacuation unnecessary.

If fluid replacement is required during evacuation, a gravity fed intravenous drip will be difficult to maintain. There are various pressure and power infusers that can be packaged with the patient, eliminating the need to hang the fluid bag above the litter. Another option is to use periodic bolus infusions administered while the litter team is taking a rest. This can be accomplished through a heparin lock or an intact system with the IV line closed while the patient is being carried. Aggressive fluid replacement for shock from severe internal bleeding can be dangerous when surgical care is not immediately available. The increase in blood pressure with volume expansion may dislodge clots causing bleeding to become worse and too much fluid can dilute clotting factors. Considering its weight versus its potential for benefit, carrying normal saline or lactated Ringers into the backcountry is usually justified only when responding to a situation where shock caused by dehydration is *likely to be on the problems list.*

(see erratum)

Section VIII

Tables and Glossary

Tables

Temperature: Fahrenheit to Celsius

°F	°C
107.6	42
105.8	41
104	40
102.2	39
100.4	38
98.6	37
95	35
89.6	32
87.8	31
86	30
84.2	29
82.4	28
68	20
59	15
50	10
41	5

Centimeters to Inches

Centimeters	Inches
1	0.393
5	1.968
10	3.937
50	19.685
100	39.370

Knots to Miles per Hour

Knots	MPH
1	1.150
5	5.753
10	11.507
15	17.261
20	23.015
25	28.769
30	34.523

Kilometers to Miles

Kilometers	Miles
1	0.621
5	3.106
10	6.213
50	31.068
100	62.137

Miles per Hour to Meters per Second

MPH	MPS
1	0.447
5	2.235
10	4.470
15	6.705
20	8.940
25	11.176
30	13.411

Kilograms to Pounds

Kilograms	Pounds
1	2.204
20	44.092
40	88.184
60	132.277
80	176.369
100	220.462
120	264.554
140	308.647

Ounces to Milliliters

Ounces	Ml
1	29.57
8	236.58
33.81	1000

GLASGOW COMA SCALE

Eye Opening Response

- Spontaneous—open with blinking at baseline 4 points

- To verbal stimuli, command, speech 3 points

- To pain only (not applied to face) 2 points

- No response 1 point

Verbal Response

- Oriented 5 points

- Confused conversation, but able to answer questions 4 points

- Inappropriate words 3 points

- Incomprehensible speech 2 points

- No response 1 point

Motor Response

- Obeys commands for movement 6 points

- Purposeful movement to painful stimulus 5 points

- Withdraws in response to pain 4 points

- Flexion in response to pain (decorticate posturing) 3 points

- Extension response in response to pain (decerebrate posturing) 2 points

- No response 1 point

Abbreviations, Acronyms and Mnemonics

A: Problem List (part of SOAP)

A': Anticipated Problem (part of SOAP)

A and O Awake and oriented

AED Automated External Defibulator

AGE Arterial Gas Embolus

APAP Acetaminophen

AVPU Awake
Verbal stimulus response
Painful stimulus response
Unresponsive

ALS Advanced Life Support

ASA Aspirin

ASR Acute Stress Reaction

BBP Blood-borne Pathogen

BLS Basic Life Support

BSA Body Surface Area

c With

CC Chief Complaint

C/MS Level of Consciousness and Mental Status

CNS Central Nervous System
c/o Complains of

CPR Cardiopulmonary Resuscitation

CSM Circulation, Sensation, and Movement

CVA Cerebro-Vascular Accident (stroke)

D50 Dextrose-50 (sugar solution)

EMS Emergency Medical Services

EMT Emergency Medical Technician

ETOH Ethanol (Alcohol)

GI Gastrointestinal

HACE High Altitude Cerebral Edema

HAPE High Altitude Pulmonary Edema

Hx History

IC Incident Commander

ICP Intracranial Pressure

ICS Incident Command System

IM Intramuscular

IV Intravenous

mcg microgram; 1/1000 of a milligram

MDI Metered Dose Inhaler

mg milligram; 1/1000 of a gram

mmol.L millimoles per liter

MI   Myocardial Infarction (heart attack)

MOI   Mechanism of Injury

M/S   Mental Status

NP   Nurse Practitioner

NPO   Nothing by Mouth. From the latin nil per os.

NSAIDs Non-Steroidal Anti-inflammatory Drugs

O: Objective (part of SOAP)

O2   Oxygen

OM   otitis media; Ear Infection

P: Plan (part of SOAP)

PA   Physician Assistant

PAS   Patient Assessment System

PCN   Penicillin

PEP   Post Exposure Prophylaxis

PFA   Pain-Free Activity

po   per os; By Mouth

PPV   Positive Pressure Ventilation

pr   per rectum

PROP Position
        Reassurance
        Oxygen
        Positive Pressure Ventilation

prn   as needed

qd   each day

q4h   every 4 hours

RF   Red Flag

RICE Rest
        Ice
        Compression
        Elevation

Rx   Treatment or prescription

S: Subjective

SAMPLE Symptoms
        Allergies
        Medicines
        Past history of medical problems
        Last meal
        Events leading up to injury

s   without

sc   subcutaneous; under the skin

sl   sub lingual; under the tongue

SOB   Shortness of Breath

SOAP   Subjective - Information gained by
             questioning
           Objective - Information gathered during
             examination of the patient
           Assessment - List of problems discovered
           Plan - What is to be done about each
             problem

STOPEATS
    Sugar
    Temperature
    Oxygen
    Pressure
    Electricity
    Altitude
    Toxins
    Salts

sx   Symptoms

s/sx   Signs and symptoms

TBI   Traumatic Brain Injury

TIP   Traction into Position

TM   Tympanic Membrane; Ear Drum

VS   Vital Signs (with time recorded)
        BP - Blood Pressure
        R - Respiratory Rate
        T - Core Temperature
        C - Level of Consciousness (Mental
           Status if Awake)
        S - Skin
        P - Pulse

WALS® Wilderness Advanced Life Support

WARM Wilderness and Rescue Medicine

WBLS Wilderness Basic Life Support

WEMR Wilderness Emergency Medical Responder

WEMT Wilderness Emergency Medical Technician

WFR   Wilderness First Responder

WMA   Wilderness Medical Associates

Glossary

Abrasion: Superficial wound that damages only the outermost layers of skin or cornea.

Abscess: A localized infection isolated from the rest of the body by inflammation.

Acute Stress Reaction (ASR): Autonomic nervous system controlled response to stress that can cause severe but temporary and reversible changes in vital signs.

Advanced Life Support: The emergency treatment of major critical system problems using medications and advanced procedures.

Airway: The passage for air exchange between the alveoli of the lungs and the outside. Most commonly refers to the upper airway, including the nose, mouth, and trachea.

Alkalosis: Abnormal drop in acidity of the blood. Can be caused by a decrease in carbon dioxide in the blood or by certain toxins.

Altitude Illness: The constellation of symptoms produced by altitude adjustment, high altitude cerebral edema, and high altitude pulmonary edema. Can be mild, moderate, or severe.

Alveoli: Membranous air sacks in the lungs where gas is exchanged with the blood.

Amnesia: Loss of memory.

Anaphylaxis: Systemic allergic reaction involving generalized edema of all body surfaces, vascular shock, and respiratory distress.

Angina: The pain of myocardial ischemia. Also called *Angina pectoris*. May be stable or unstable.

Antibiotic: A drug that selectively kills or interferes with the function or reproduction of bacteria.

Anticipated Problems (A'): Problems that may develop over time as a result of injury, illness, or the environment.

Antifungal: A drug that selectively kills or interferes with the function or reproduction of pathogenic fungus.

Antiviral: A drug that selectively kills or interferes with the function or reproduction of viruses.

Arrhythmia: Abnormal heart rhythm. Also called a *dysrhythmia*.

Artery: Vessel carrying blood from the heart to the capillary beds in body tissues. Arteries have muscular walls, the constriction of which contribute to maintaining perfusion pressure. Carries blood under high pressure.

Aspiration: Inhaling foreign liquid or other material into the lungs.

Ataxia: Stumbling gait.

Basic Life Support (BLS): The generic process of supporting the functions of the circulatory, respiratory, and nervous systems using CPR, bleeding control, and spine stabilization.

Beta-agonist: Drug that stimulates beta-adrenergic receptors in body cells. This is used primarily to relax the smooth muscle lining the bronchial tubes in the treatment of asthma and other causes of lower airway constriction. Examples include albuterol, salmeterol, and metaproterenol.

Biphasic Reaction: Return of the symptoms of anaphylaxis after treatment caused by the continued presence of the antigen, and the metabolism and excretion of the emergency medications.

Blood Pressure Cuff: Also known as a *sphygmomanometer*. Used for measuring blood pressure.

Bronchospasm: Contraction of the muscular walls of the bronchial tubes.

Bronchi and Bronchioles: Tubes of the lower airway conducting air to the alveoli of the lungs.

Capillaries: The smallest blood vessels in body tissues where gasses and nutrients are exchanged between tissue cells and the circulating blood.

Cardiac arrest: Loss of effective heart activity.

Cardiogenic Shock: Shock due to inadequate pumping action of the heart.

Cardiopulmonary Resuscitation (CPR): A technique for artificially circulating oxygenated blood in the absence of effective heart activity. Includes positive pressure ventilation (PPV) and chest compressions.

Carotid Pulse: The pulse felt on the side of the neck at the site of the carotid artery.

Cartilage: Connective tissue on the ends of bones at joints that provides a smooth gliding surface.

Central Nervous System: The brain and spinal cord.

Cervical Spine: The section of the spine in the neck between the base of the skull and the top of the thorax.

Clotting Factors: Chemicals in the blood contributing to the process of blood clotting.

Cold Challenge: The combined cooling influence of wind, humidity, and ambient temperature.

Cold Diuresis: Increased urination resulting from the shell core effect in cold response and hypothermia.

Cold Response: The normal body response to the cold challenge, including shell/core effect and shivering.

Compartment Syndrome: Swelling within a confined body compartment, like the connective tissue compartments in the leg or inside the skull, that results in ischemia.

Compensation: Involuntary changes in body functions designed to maintain perfusion pressure and oxygenation of vital body tissues in the presence of injury or illness.

Concussion: Brain injury. May be mild or severe. Also called *head injury* or *traumatic brain injury.*

Conjunctiva: The membrane covering the white of the eye and the inner surfaces of the eye lids.

Conjunctivitis: Inflammation of the conjunctiva due to irritation, infection, or injury. Most often used in reference to infection (pink eye).

Contusion: Bruise or blunt injury to bone or soft tissue.

Cornea: The clear part of the eye over the iris and pupil.

Cornice: An overhanging drift of snow formed as wind blows over a ridge or mountaintop.

Crepitis: The feel or sound of bones or cartilage grating when moved. Typical at the site of an unstable fracture. Can also describe the feel or sound of subcutaneous air when palpated.

Cyanosis: The blue color seen in the lips and skin of a patient with poor tissue oxygenation. This is actually the color of de-oxygenated hemoglobin.

Debridement: Wound cleaning, including removal of foreign material and devitalized tissue.

Definitive Medical Care: Therapy that cures the disease or corrects the problem.

Dental Abscess: Infection at the base of a tooth.

Diagnosis: The identification of a medical problem by name. May be generic or specific.

Diaphragm: Muscle at the lower end of the chest cavity, which contracts to create a vacuum that draws air into the lungs. The diaphragm works with muscles of the chest wall, shoulders, and neck to perform ventilation.

Diastolic Blood Pressure: The standing pressure within the circulatory system remaining while the heart is between contractions. Documented as the second or lower number in blood pressure.

Differential Diagnosis: The list of possible causes of a medical problem or symptom.

Dilutional Hypotremia: Condition of electrolyte dilution caused by excessive water intake.

Discharge: Fluid escaping from the site of infection or inflammation. Also called exudate.

Dislocation: Disruption of normal joint anatomy.

Distal: An anatomical direction; away from the body center. The wrist is distal to the elbow.

Dura: Connective tissue and membrane lining of the cranium and brain.

Dyspnea: Also called shortness of breath, respiratory distress, or difficulty breathing.

Dysrhythmia: An abnormal heart rhythm. Also called arrhythmia.

Edema: Swelling due to leaking of serum from capillaries.

Electrolyte: Elements or molecules in the blood. Examples include sodium, potassium, chloride, and calcium.

Embolus: Object or substance traveling in the blood capable of lodging in the circulatory system and causing ischemia. Examples include bubbles of air, fat globules, and freely floating blood clots.

Emphysema: Chronic lower airway constriction leading to lung hyperinflation and the formation of cavities within lung tissue.

Epinephrine: The synthetic form of the hormone adrenalin. Used to constrict blood vessels and dilate airway tubes.

EpiPen®: Device that automatically injects 0.3 mg of epinephrine when armed and triggered.

Evacuation: Transferring a patient from the scene of injury or illness to definitive medical care.

Eviceration: Injury that leaves abdominal or thoracic organs outside the body.

Exertional Hyponatremia: Condition of electrolyte dilution caused by loss of body salts due to excessive sweating.

Extension: Movement at a joint that extends an extremity away from the center of the body. The opposite of flexion.

Extracellular space: Between and among the cells of body tissues.

Extrication: Removing or freeing a patient from entrapment or confinement.

Exudate: Discharge, usually from a wound or infection.

Fascia: Layer of tough connective tissue separating and supporting layers of soft tissue.

Femoral Artery: Large artery that travels along the femur in the thigh.

Femur: Long bone of the thigh.

Flail Chest: The loss of rigidity of the chest wall due to multiple rib fractures.

Flexion: Movement of a joint that brings the extremity closer to the body. The opposite of extension.

Focused History and Physical Exam: The third stage in the patient assessment system; includes the examination of the whole body, SAMPLE History, and Vital Signs.

Fracture: Broken bone, cartilage, or solid organ.

Frostbite: Frozen tissue. May be partial thickness or deep.

Frostnip: Loss of circulation due to the vasoconstriction of blood vessels in the skin during the early stages of tissue freezing. Also called *superficial frostbite.*

Glaucoma: Disease or condition causing increased pressure within the globe of the eye.

Glycogen: Carbohydrate stored in the liver and muscles. Glycogen is converted into sugar for use as fuel during exercise.

Head Injury: Injury to the brain. Also called *concussion.*

Heart Attack: Heart muscle ischemia caused by a blood clot or spasm of the coronary arteries or by an arrhythmia, resulting in the necrosis (or infarction) of heart tissue.

Heat Challenge: Combined effects of ambient temperature and metabolic activity that contribute to body heating.

Heat Exhaustion: Compensated volume shock caused by fluid loss due to sweating.

Heat Response: The normal body response to the heat challenge, including sweating and vasodilation of the shell.

Heat Stroke: Severe elevation of body temperature (over 105° F).

Hemoglobin: Molecule contained within red blood cells that binds to oxygen during its transport to body cells.

Hemothorax: Blood in the chest cavity as a result of injury, usually collecting between the chest wall and lung tissue.

Hollow Organs: The stomach, intestines, bladder and other organs enclosing space occupied by fluid and/or gas.

Hormones: Chemical compounds released by glands to have specific effects of specific body tissues.

Histamine: Hormone released by various processes causing, among other effects, vasodilation and bronchoconstriction.

Hyperextension: To extend a joint beyond its normal range of motion.

Hyperventilation syndrome: Respiratory alkalosis. The nervous system symptoms of numbness, visual field contraction, and light-headedness caused by reduced carbon dioxide in the blood due to excessive ventilation, usually associated with acute stress reaction .

Hypoglycemia: Low blood sugar.

Hypothermia: Below normal body core temperature (37°C).

Hypoxia: Lack of oxygen.

Infarction: Tissue death due to loss of oxygenation and perfusion. Also called necrosis.

Infection: Pathologic colonization of body tissues by bacteria, virus, fungus, or other micro-organisms.

Inflammation: A generic body response to illness or injury resulting in redness, swelling, warmth, and tenderness.

Initial Assessment: The second stage of the patient assessment system and the initial examination of the patient. Looks for life-threatening problems with the critical functions of the circulatory, respiratory, and nervous systems.

Intoxication: Altered level of consciousness or mental status due to the influence of chemicals such as drugs, alcohol, and inhaled gasses.

Intracellular space: Inside the cells of body tissues.

Intracranial: Inside the skull (cranium).

Intravenous Fluids: Fluids infused directly into the circulatory system through a hypodermic needle inserted into a vein, usually used to temporarily increase the volume of circulating blood or restore fluid lost to sweating or diarrhea.

Intubation: Placing an endotrachial tube or Combitube device into the trachea.

Involuntary Guarding: Refers to abdominal muscle spasm to protect the abdomen from painful movement. Considered a sign of peritoneal irritation.

Ischemia: Lack of local perfusion to body tissues. Can be caused by a clot, constriction, shell/core effect, or tight splint. Persistent ischemia will result in infarction.

Level of Consciousness: Describes the level of brain function in terms of responsiveness to specific stimuli: (The AVPU Scale) **A** = Awake, **V** = responds to Verbal stimuli, **P** = responds to Painful stimuli, **U** = Unresponsive to any stimuli.

Ligaments: Tough connective tissue joining bone to bone across joints.

Local Effects: Effects that are restricted to the immediate area of injury or infection (versus systemic effects).

Long Bones: Bones that have a long structural axis such as leg and arm bones as opposed to flat bones such as ribs and shoulder blades.

Lower Airway: trachea, bronchi, and alveoli.

Lumbar Spine: The lower section of the spine between the thorax and the pelvis.

Lymphangitis: Spread of a local infection into the lymph system. The early stage of a systemic infection. Symptoms include red streaks running centrally from the site of a local infection.

Mechanism of Injury (MOI): The cause of injury or a description of the forces involved.

Mental Status: Describes the level of brain function in an awake patient (A on AVPU) in terms of memory, orientation, level of anxiety, and behavior.

Mid-Range Position: Position in a joint's range of motion between full extension and full flexion. Also called *neutral position.*

Neurovascular Bundle: An artery, vein, and nerve combination routed though the body together

Neutral position: The position approximately half way between flexion and extension. Also called the *mid-range position.*

Normal Saline: A fluid used for volume replacement or wound irrigation having the same percentage of salt as the blood and body tissues.

Open Fracture: Fracture with an associated break in the skin. Also called a compound fracture.

Oxygenation: To saturate blood with oxygen in the lungs. Also describes the transfer of oxygen from the blood to body cells (cellular oxygenation).

Parasthesia: Neurological deficit, usually described as weakness or numbness and tingling.

Patella: Knee cap.

Pathologic: Harmful to the body. Usually used to describe bacteria, fungus, or virus.

Patient Assessment System: A system of surveys including Scene Size-Up, Primary Survey, and Secondary Survey designed to gather information about an injured or ill patient and the environment in which the patient is found.

Percussion: Examination technique using tapping to elicit tenderness or sounds. For example, tapping teeth gently with a stick to elicit tenderness or percussing the abdomen to evaluate distention.

Perfusion: The passage of blood through capillary beds in body tissues.

Peristalsis: The wave of muscular contraction in the stomach and intestine used to move food and fluid.

Peripheral Nerves: The nerves running between body tissues and the spinal cord.

Peritoneal Signs: Signs and symptoms caused by irritation of the peritoneal lining of the abdomen and pelvis.

Photophobia: Eye pain or headache caused by bright lights.

Plasma: The liquid portion of the blood consisting of water, proteins, and other compounds.

Pneumonia: Infection of lung tissue resulting in the accumulation of fluid in the alveoli.

Pneumothorax: Free air in the chest cavity, usually from a punctured lung or chest wall.

Polypro: Slang for polypropylene clothing.

Post Concussive Syndrome: Various symptoms following impact injury to the head. Includes anorexia, photophobia, lethargy, and irritability.

Posturing: Global extensor or flexor muscle contraction resulting from severe brain injury. An indication of severe increased intracranial pressure.

Problem List: Assessment. The list of problems identified by the Patient Assessment System.

Prophylaxis: Treatment initiated to prevent a problem from developing. For example, prophylactic antibiotics to prevent infection in high-risk wounds.

Proximal: Toward the center of the body. The elbow is proximal to the wrist.

Pulmonary Edema: Swelling of lung tissue resulting in the collection of fluid in the alveoli.

Pulse Oximeter: Device that measures the percentage of hemoglobin in the blood that is saturated with oxygen.

Rales: Fine crackles. The noise produced by pulmonary edema. Sounds like crinkling cellophane or air being sucked through a wet sponge.

Reduction: Restoring a dislocated joint to normal position. Also restoring a displaced fracture to normal anatomic position.

Red Blood Cells: Cells floating in the blood that contain hemoglobin. Primarily responsible for carrying oxygen.

Rhabdomyalasis: A condition in which the breakdown of damaged and ischemic muscle cells release myoglobin, enzymes, and electrolytes that can cause kidney failure.

Rhonchi: Coarse crackles. The sound produced by mucous or fluid in the lower airways.

Rule out: Used as a verb for the act of determining that a condition or problem does not exist.

Scene Size-Up: The first stage of the patient assessment system during which you look for dangers to the rescuer and patient, numbers of people injured, and the mechanism of injury.

Seizure: Uncoordinated electrical activity in the brain.

Sepsis: Systemic infection.

Serum: The liquid portion of the blood, as distinguished from blood cells and platelets.

Sexually Transmitted Disease (STD): Infection transmitted from person to person by sexual activity.

Shell/Core Compensation: Vasoconstriction in the skin and gut to shunt blood to vital body organs. Occurs as a result of volume shock and cold response.

Shell/Core Effect: A compensation mechanism seen in shock and cold response that reduces blood flow to the body shell in order to preserve perfusion and warmth in the vital organs of the core. Can also be reversed in core/shell effect.

Shock: Inadequate perfusion pressure in the circulatory system resulting in inadequate cellular oxygenation.

Signs: Response elicited by examination, e.g., pain when the examiner touches an injured area (tenderness).

Sinus: Hollow spaces in the bones of the skull.

Sinusitis: Inflammation of the membranous lining of the sinuses due to infection, allergy, or toxic exposure. Usually used in reference to infection.

Solid Organs: Liver, spleen, pancreas, kidneys and other organs without significant hollow space.

Spasm: Involuntary contraction of muscle.

Spinal Cord: The cord-like extension of the central nervous system encased within the bones of the spinal column, running from the base of the brain to the mid-lumbar spine.

Spine: The column of bony vertebrae extending from the base of the skull to the pelvis. Includes the bones, ligaments, cartilage, and spinal cord.

Spine Assessment: A systematic examination of the spinal column and spinal cord function looking for evidence of injury.

Static rope: A rope with very limited stretch. Often used in rescue work. In contrast to a dynamic rope that has the ability to stretch and absorb shock-loading.

Stethoscope: An instrument use to transmit body sounds directly to the ears of the examiner via rubber tubes.

Stridor: Stuttering and gasping sounds made by inhalation against an upper airway obstruction.

Stroke: Localized brain ischemia caused by an embolis, clot, or blood vessel rupture.

Sub-lingual: Under the tongue. Usually refers to a route of medication administration such as a sub-lingual tablet of nitroglycerine or morphine.

Submersion Injury: At least temporary survival of water inhalation.

Survey: A systematic examination of the scene or patient.

Swelling: Abnormal fluid accumulation in body tissues due to bleeding or edema.

Symptomatic Treatment: Therapy that relieves symptoms, but does not necessarily treat the cause.

Symptoms: Conditions described by the patient, e.g., pain on swallowing.

Synovial Fluid: Joint fluid, lubrication inside a joint.

Systemic: Involving the entire body such as a systemic infection or systemic allergy.

Systolic Blood Pressure: The pressure within the circulatory system generated by contraction of the heart.

Tamponade: Bleeding within a confined space such that blood loss stops when the space if full.

Tendon: Fibrous tissue connecting muscle to bone.

Tetanus: Nervous system spasm and paralysis cause by the toxin released by *Clostridium tetani* bacteria. Also called *lock jaw*.

Thorax: The chest or chest cavity.

Tourniquet: A constricting band used to prevent or restrict the flow of blood to an extremity.

Toxin: Chemical that has a damaging effect on body tissues or the function of the nervous system.

Toxin Load: The combined systemic effect of numerous small toxic exposures such as a large number of insect bites or man-of-war stings.

Traction: Tension applied along the long axis of an extremity.

Traction Splint: A splinting device designed to maintain traction on an extremity, primarily used for femur fractures in the field setting.

Trauma: Injury.

Traumatic Brain Injury: Injury to the brain. Also called *head injury* or *concussion*.

Trench Foot: Inflammation due to ischemia and necrosis caused by cold-induced vasoconstriction during prolonged exposure to cold and wet conditions.

TwinJect™: Device that automatically injects 0.3 mg of epinephrine when armed and triggered. Also contains a second dose that is manually injected as needed.

Umbilicus: Navel, belly button.

Universal Precautions: Set of precautions or procedures to minimize the risk of disease transmission via contact with infected body fluids. Includes gloves, eye protection, face shields or masks, protective clothing, and the use of disinfectants. Universal precautions also includes proper procedures for handling and disposal of contaminated articles and instruments.

Upper Airway: Mouth, nose, throat (larynx).

Vacuum Mattress: A patient stabilization device consisting of a vinyl bag filled with plastic beads that coalesce to form a rigid package when the air is evacuated from the device.

Vapor Barrier: A vapor proof wrap or covering that prevents evaporative cooling.

Vascular Bundle: A grouped nerve, artery, and vein following the same pathway.

Vascular Shock: Shock due to dilation of blood vessels.

Vascular Space: Inside the blood vessels.

Vasodilation: Dilation of blood vessels.

Vasodilator: A drug that stimulates blood vessel dilation.

Vein: Vessel returning blood from body tissues to the heart. Equipped with one way valves to enhance flow. Carries blood under low pressure.

Ventilation: The movement of air in and out of the lungs.

Ventricular Fibrillation: Uncoordinated contraction of heart muscle. An example of a dysrhythmia.

Vertebrae: The bones of the spine.

Vital Signs: Measurements of body function including Blood Pressure, Pulse, Respiration, Level of Consciousness, Skin color, and body core Temperature.

Volume Shock: Inadequate blood volume resulting in inadequate perfusion pressure in the circulatory system leading to inadequate cellular oxygenation.

Voluntary Guarding: Voluntary contraction of abdominal muscle as the patient protects himself from the pain caused by palpation.

Wilderness Context: A situation where access to definitive medical care is delayed by distance, logistics, or danger.

Example Medications

Acetaminophen (Tylenol®, Panadol®, Paracetamol, APAP): Non-narcotic for pain and fever.
   Advantages: Inexpensive, well-known, well tolerated, very effective for pain and fever.
   Disadvantage: Does not reduce inflammation; potential liver toxicity with continued excessive doses, especially with liver disease or sustained alcohol use.
   Use: General pain reliever, fever reducer. Not useful for swelling.
   Side Effects: Infrequent. Causes less stomach upset than ibuprofen.
   Precautions: Hypersensitivity to acetaminophen.
   Administration: One to two 325 mg tablets every 4–6 hours or two 500 mg tablets every 6 hours as needed. May be given in alternating doses with ibuprofen to increase pain relief and reduce inflammation.

Acetaminophen with oxycodone (Percocet®): combined non-narcotic analgesic and narcotic pain reliever. Rx.
   Advantages: Inexpensive. Good pain relief spectrum. Can be combined with ibuprofen.
   Disadvantages: Side effects of narcotics. Street value. Controlled substance.
   Use: Moderate to severe pain.
   Side Effects: Drowsiness, slow reaction time, occasional stomach upset. Will cause constipation—give plenty of fiber and water.
   Precautions: Hypersensitivity to Tylenol® or oxycodone. Use with caution in situations where patient must remain alert. Do not give with additional Tylenol®.
   Administration: One tablet every 6 hours for pain. May be given in alternating doses with ibuprofen to increase pain relief and reduce inflammation. Supplied in various strengths; 7.5/500, for example, indicates 7.5 mg of oxycodone and 500 mg of APAP.

Albuterol (Ventolin®) metered dose inhaler: inhaled bronchodilator. Rx.
   Advantages: Easy to use and carry. Inexpensive.
   Disadvantages: Easy to overuse.
   Use: Reverse bronchospasm and reduce wheezing in asthma and bronchitis.
   Side Effects: Nausea, palpitations, nervousness, high blood pressure.
   Precautions: Hypersensitivity to albuterol. Albuterol, as with all sympathomimetic amines, should be used with caution in patients with cardiovascular disorders, especially coronary insufficiency, cardiac arrhythmias, and hypertension; in patients with convulsive disorders, hyperthyroidism, or diabetes mellitus; and in patients who are unusually responsive to sympathomimetic amines. Clinically significant changes in systolic and diastolic blood pressure have been seen and could be expected to occur in some patients after use of any beta-adrenergic bronchodilator.
   Administration: Up to two inhalations every 4 - 6 hours for relief of mild to moderate symptoms. Do not exceed recommended dose except in emergency. It is recommended to test spray inhalation aerosol into the air before using for the first time and in cases where the aerosol has not been used for a prolonged period of time. For emergency use in severe asthma following epinephrine treatment; may give up to 6–10 puffs three times over next hour. See asthma protocols.

Azithromycin (Zithromax®): macrolide antibiotic. Rx.
    Advantages: Effective, easy dosage, and short course of therapy.
    Disadvantages: Expensive.
    Use: Bronchitis, pneumonia, uncomplicated skin infections, pharyngitis, tonsillitis, ear infection, sinus infection. Can also be used to treat chlamydia and gonococcal urethritis. Also indicated for travelers' diarrhea.
    Precautions: Hypersensitivity to macrolides including erythromycin.
    Side Effects: Usually limited to diarrhea and stomach upset. Not frequent.
    Administration: Take 2 tablets on the first day, then 1 each day for next 4 days. Tablets may be taken without food. Also available as 500 mg tablets to be taken once per day for 3 days. A single dose of 1 gram may be used to treat some conditions, particularly sexually transmitted diseases. A single dose of 250 mg may be used to treat uncomplicated travelers' diarrhea.

Bisacodyl suppositories and tablets (Dulcolax®): laxative, rectal stimulant.
    Use: Laxative
    Side Effects: Abdominal pain and cramping.
    Precautions: Do not use oral laxative products when abdominal pain, nausea, or vomiting are present unless directed by a physician. If you have noticed a sudden change in bowel habits that persists over a period of 2 weeks, consult a physician before using a laxative. Restoration of normal bowel function by using this product may cause abdominal discomfort, including cramps. Laxative products should not be used for a period longer than 1 week unless directed by a physician. Rectal bleeding or failure to have a bowel movement after use of a laxative may indicate a serious condition. If this occurs, discontinue use and consult your physician.
    Administration: Adults and children 12 years of age and over: 1 suppository once daily. Remove foil wrapper. Lie on your side and, with pointed end first, push suppository high into the rectum so it will not slip out. Retain it for 15–20 minutes. If you feel the suppository must come out immediately, it was not inserted high enough and should be pushed higher. Children 6–12 years of age: ½ suppository. Expect results in 8–12 hours if taken at bedtime or within 6 hours if taken before breakfast.

Cephalexin (Keflex®, Keftab®): cephalosporin antibiotic. Rx.
    Advantages: Well-known, broad spectrum, effective, inexpensive.
    Disadvantages: Four times a day dosing.
    Use: Skin and bone infections, prophylaxis in high-risk wounds like bites, deep or very dirty wounds, and open fractures. Can also be used for respiratory infections, urinary tract infections, ear infections.
    Precautions: Hypersensitivity to cephalosprorins. There is a 10% cross-reactivity with penicillin allergy.
    Side Effects: Usually limited to diarrhea and stomach upset. Not frequent.
    Administration: For serious infections, give two 500 mg capsules every 6 hours, usually for 7 days (2 grams/day). For less serious infections, give one 250 mg capsule every 6 hours for 7 days.

Ceftriaxone (Rocephin® vials for injection): 3rd generation cepholosporin antibiotic. Rx.
    Advantages: Broad spectrum, IM or IV dosing once or twice a day.
    Disadvantages: Very expensive, injection is painful.
    Use: Severe infections. Pelvic inflammatory disease, intra-abdominal infections. Joint infections, infections not responding to oral antibiotics.

Side Effects: Infrequent, usually limited to diarrhea.

Precautions: Hypersensitivity to cepholosporins.

Administration: Give 1 gram every 24 hours. May increase to 1 gram every 12 hours in severe infections. Using a 3 cc syringe and a 22 x 1.5" needle, inject two ml of 1% plain lidocaine into the vial and shake until powder is completely dissolved. Draw suspension back into the syringe and inject deep intramuscular (outer, upper quadrant of buttocks).

Ciprofloxacin (Cipro® 500 mg tablets): fluoroquinolone antibiotic. Rx.

Advantages: Broad spectrum, covers marine pathogens and pseudomonas.

Disadvantages: Expensive, does not cover some staph and strep very well.

Use: Urinary tract infections, skin and soft tissue infections—particularly where contamination from rubber boots or wet suits is involved—or in wounds exposed to salt water. Sinusitis. Can also be used for prostatitis, respiratory infections, intra-abdominal infections.

Precautions: Hypersensitivity to "floxins." Can cause photosensivity—avoid unprotected exposure to sunlight.

Side Effects: Diarrhea, stomach upset, agitation, insomnia, tendon injury.

Administration: For travelers' diarrhea, give one 750 mg tablet every day for up to 3 days. One dose may do it. Otherwise, generally for use when other antibiotics have been ineffective. Give one 750 mg tablet every 12 hours with or without food.

Cortisporin otic suspension: combination antibiotic for external ear. Rx.

Use: Swimmer's ear, evidenced by swollen, tender ear canal.

Side Effects: Infrequent, usually increased irritation caused by sensitivity to Neomycin.

Precautions: Hypersensitivity to mycins, polymixin, or hydrocortisone. Prolonged use may cause overgrowth of nonsensitive bacteria. Do not use as a preventive.

Administration: Clean ear canal with cotton swab. Have patient lie down with affected ear up. Instill 4–5 drops in the ear and have patient remain in place for about 30 minutes. Give 2–3 times a day for 1 full day following clearing of symptoms.

Diphenhydramine 25 mg capsules (Benadryl®): antihistamine H1.

Advantages: Inexpensive, generic, well-known, generally well-tolerated, wide spectrum of activity and use.

Disadvantages: Causes drowsiness in therapeutic dosages.

Use: Allergy and anaphylaxis. Itching. Nasal and sinus congestion. Nausea. Sea sickness. Insomnia. Anxiety.

Side Effects: Primarily drowsiness. Can cause urinary retention in patients with prostate enlargement.

Precautions: May cause marked drowsiness; alcohol, sedatives, and tranquilizers may increase the drowsiness effect. Avoid alcoholic beverages while taking this product. Do not take this product if you are taking sedatives or tranquilizers, without first consulting your doctor. Use caution when driving a motor vehicle or operating machinery. **Do not use any other products containing diphenhydramine while using this product.**

Administration: 25–50 mg every 6 hours.

Epinephrine 1:1000 solution: vasoconstrictor, bronchodilator. Rx.

Advantages: Inexpensive, life-saving drug for anaphylaxis and asthma.

Disadvantages: Expensive when supplied in an EpiPen® or TwinJect™ Autoinjector. Short shelf life.

Use: Emergency treatment of anaphylaxis and severe asthma. Followed by diphenhydramine and prednisone (or Medrol dose pack). See anaphylaxis and asthma protocols.

Side Effects: Agitation, tachycardia.

Precautions: Can cause heart attack to become worse (but, so can anaphylaxis and asthma). Can elevate blood pressure. Be confident of your diagnosis before injecting this medication.

Administration: For anaphylaxis give 0.3 mg epinephrine IM or SC. Follow immediately by 50 mg of diphenhydramine orally or IM, and 20–60 mg (depending on body weight) of prednisone orally for anaphylaxis. Epinephrine may be repeated every 5 minutes if necessary if improvement is slow or rebound reaction occurs. For severe asthma when albuterol inhaler is not working, give same dose of epinephrine and prednisone as for anaphylaxis. Diphenhydramine is not necessary or useful for asthma. See asthma and anaphylaxis protocols.

Famotidine (Pepcid®): antihistamine H2 blocker.

Advantages: Inexpensive, non-prescription.

Disadvantages: No real disadvantage.

Use: Gastric acid problems; reflux, esophagitis, ulcer. Because it is an antihistamine covering different receptors, Pepcid can also be used as an adjunct in the treatment of anaphylaxis or allergic rash not responding well to diphenhydramine. This can be particularly useful for recalcitrant urticaria (e.g., hives).

Side Effects: Headache, dizziness, constipation, diarrhea.

Precautions: Allergy to antihistamines.

Administration: 20 mg every 12–24 hours as needed to reduce symptoms. Higher doses may be given to control ulcers, but should be done with medical advice.

Fentanyl (Actiq®): narcotic analgesic. Rx.

Advantages: Fentanyl is a potent narcotic analgesic available for IV, IM, or transmucosal administration. It is less prone to cause nausea than morphine, and is very short acting. The transmucosal "fentanyl pop" (Actiq®) offers an attractive option for use in remote and extreme environments where the use of IV and IM medications is difficult. The medication is held in the mouth by the patient, who can self-regulate the amount of pain medication desired during extrication or painful procedures like shoulder reduction. Anecdotally, military units report considerable success with fentanyl transmucosal pops with combat casualties using the 400 microgram dose.

Disadvantages: Atiq transmucosal fentanyl is generally sold only for breakthrough cancer pain and may be difficult to obtain for other purposes. Don't expect your practitioner to be comfortable prescribing fentanyl unless she or he has experience with it. Street value. Expensive.

Use: "Pops" for short-term patient-regulated pain control.

Side Effects: Drowsiness, slow reaction time, constipation, impaired respiration if combined with other narcotics or given in too high a dose.

Precautions: Can cause respiratory depression. Increase dose carefully. Be ready to provide ventilations if necessary. Pop can cause airway obstruction—monitor the patient at all times. Best given under medical supervision or advice.

Administration: Consider Actiq transmucosal pops in 200 or 400 microgram doses. Specific instructions for use should be given by the prescribing practitioner.

Fluconazole (Diflucan® 150 mg tablets): antifungal for vaginal yeast infections. Rx.
Advantages: One tablet treats the infection.
Disadvantages: Prescription medication, expensive. High incidence of drug interactions. If on other meds, seek medical advice before using.
Use: Vaginal yeast infections.
Side Effects: Headache, nausea, abdominal pain. Generally transient and not serious.
Precautions: Will not treat bacterial vaginoses. Hypersensitivity to fluconazole.
Administration: A single one-tablet dose by mouth.

Glucagon: converts hepatic glycogen to glucose. Rx.
Use: Emergency treatment of severe hypoglycemia.
Side Effects: Hypotension, nausea, vomiting, urticaria, respiratory distress, hyperglycemia.
Administration: 0.5–1 mg given IV, IM, or SC. May repeat in 25 minutes.

Ibuprofen (Motrin®, Advil®): NSAID for pain, fever, and inflammation.
Advantages: Inexpensive, well-known, very effective for mild to moderate pain, inflammation, fever.
Disadvantages: Three times per day dosing, some people experience stomach upset.
Use: General pain reliever, reducing fever, reducing swelling in infection, injury, and sunburn.
Side Effects: Usually stomach upset.
Precautions: hypersensitivity to ibuprofen or other NSAIDs. Will increase bleeding. Can cause kidney problems in dehydrated patients.
Administration: 600 mg 6–8 hours with food and water. May be given in alternating doses with acetaminophen to increase pain relief and reduce inflammation.

Loperamide (Imodium® 2 mg capsules) : reduces gut motility for the treatment of diarrhea.
Use: diarrhea
Side Effects: Abdominal cramping, gas.
Precautions: Do not use if diarrhea is accompanied by high fever (greater than 38.5°C or 101°F) , or if blood or mucous is present in the stool, or if you have had a rash or other allergic reaction to loperamide HCL
Administration: Adults and children 12 years of age and older: Take 4 teaspoonfuls (1 dosage cup) or 2 caplets after the first loose bowel movement and 2 teaspoonfuls or 1 caplet after each subsequent loose bowel movement, but no more than 8 teaspoonfuls or 4 caplets a day for no more than 2 days. Children 9–11 years old (60–95 lbs): Take 2 teaspoonfuls (1/2 dosage cup) or 1 caplet after the first loose bowel movement and 1 teaspoonful or 1/2 caplet after each subsequent loose bowel movement but no more than 6 teaspoonfuls or 3 caplets a day for no more than 2 days. Children 6–8 years old (48–59 lbs): Take 2 teaspoonfuls (1/2 dosage cup) or 1 caplet after the first loose bowel movement and 1 teaspoonful or 1/2 caplet after each subsequent loose bowel movement but no more than 4 teaspoonfuls or 2 caplets a day for no more than 2 days.

Lorazepam (Ativan®): anxiolytic, benzodiazepine. Rx.

    Advantages: Inexpensive, well tolerated.

    Disadvantages: Street value, abuse potential.

    Use: Symptoms of acute anxiety. Useful as an adjunct to narcotics and NSAIDs in the treatment of pain.

    Side Effects: Sedation, dizziness, weakness, unsteadiness, transient amnesia, memory impairment.

    Precautions: See side effects. Avoid with primary depression or psychosis. Withdrawal symptoms with abrupt discontinuation. Can be habit forming. See full warnings in PDR.

    Administration: For anxiety 2–5 mg two or three times a day. As an adjunct to pain medication, 5–10 mg two or three times a day.

Miconazole (Monistat® 7 Vaginal Suppositories): for yeast infection.

    Advantages: Non-prescription.

    Disadvantages: Messy, melts in hot weather. Is redundant to Diflucan tablet.

    Use: Vaginal yeast infection.

    Side Effects: Minimal, irritation if hypersensitive.

    Precautions: Will not treat bacterial vaginoses. Hypersensitivity to any components.

    Administration: One suppository every day at bedtime for 3–7 days.

Mupirocin 2% (Bactroban® cream or ointment): antibiotic ointment. Rx.

    Use: An effective topical antibiotic for small secondarily infected skin lesions. Can be as effective as oral antibiotics. Can also be used in the nose to limit the recurrence of furuncles (e.g., boils)and impetigo by eliminating bacterial colonization in the nose

    Side Effects: Burning, pain, itching, headache, rash, nausea.

    Precautions: Avoid eyes. Discontinue if sensitization or irritation occurs. Avoid mucosal surfaces. Not for prolonged use.

    Administration: Apply 3 times per day for up to 10 days. May cover cream with gauze pad or bandaid. Reevaluate treatment if no response in 3–5 days.

Oxymetazalone (Afrin® Nasal Spray): vasoconstrictor, nasal decongestant.

    Use: Reduce nasal congestion, reduce equalizing problems when diving and snorkeling. Will help stop nose bleeds.

    Side Effects: Dry mouth, palpitations.

    Precautions: Do not exceed recommended dose. Do not use for more than 3 days at a time.

    Administration: One or two sprays every 12 hours.

Permethrin (Nix® Crème Rinse): topical treatment for lice.

    Use: Eradicating body and scalp lice.

    Side Effects: Hypersensitivity reactions to permetherin.

    Precautions: Hypersensitivity to permentherin.

    Administration: Apply to hair after wash and towel dry. Saturate the hair and scalp. Wash off after 10 minutes. Remove nits with the comb provided. Repeat after 7 days if live lice are observed. Use Nix spray on upholstery and bedding.

Povidone iodine solution (Betadine®) and swabsticks: topical antiseptic.

   Use: Antiseptic. Sterilize instruments and skin surfaces. Can be used to disinfect drinking water and water for irrigation.

   Side Effects: Minor skin irritation if left on for prolonged period. Kills things, including healthy skin cells if used in wounds.

   Precautions: Dilute to 1% or less for use in wounds. If used to disinfect drinking water, use a lower concentration (see below) and don't use for drinking water for more than a few weeks.   Don't use if pregnant or if there is a history of thyroid disease.

   Application: Can be used in full strength on intact skin before surgical procedures such as incising abscess or puncturing blister. Can be applied to intact skin around a wound before irrigation to avoid contamination of the wound from skin surface. Can be used to disinfect water for use as irrigation fluid or for drinking (up to 4 drops per liter of water). Can be used as a vaginal douche to treat yeast or bacterial vaginal infection (5 cc of betadine to a liter of water).

Prednisone: steroid anti-inflammatory. Rx.

   Advantages: Inexpensive, easily available.

   Disadvantages: Long-term therapy (> 5 days) will require a tapered dose calculated by the prescribing practitioner. Redundant to Medrol dose pack.

   Use: Inflammation not responding well to ibuprofen such as poison ivy, jellyfish stings. Asthma not responding to inhaler. Adjunct to the treatment of anaphylaxis and severe asthma.

   Side Effects: Stomach upset, agitation.

   Precautions: Do not use for infection unless combined with antibiotics.

   Administration: 1 mg per kilogram of body weight up to 60 mg per day for most situations. Therapy for longer than 5 days should include a tapered dose.

Pseudoephedrine (Sudafed®): decongestant, vasoconstrictor.

   Advantages: Inexpensive, well-known.

   Disadvantages: Side effects of cardiovascular stimulant. Short duration of action. Consider long acting version, timed-release capsules.

   Use: Reduces nasal and sinus congestion.

   Side Effects: Palpitations. Urinary retention. Nervousness, insomnia.

   Precautions: Do not use this product if you are now taking a prescription monoamine oxidase inhibitor or for 2 weeks after stopping the MAOI drug. If you are uncertain whether your prescription drug contains an MAOI, consult a health professional before taking this product. Avoid using if there is a history of high blood pressure.

   Administration: 30–60 mg every 6 hours. May be taken with benadryl and or ibuprofen for relief of cold and "flu" symptoms.

Senna (Senekot®): stool softener for constipation.

   Use: Bowel stimulant for constipation.

   Side Effects: Soft stool, diarrhea.

   Precautions: Will not work if constipation is caused by dehydration. Drink plenty of water.

   Administration: Two or three tablets with water.

Scopolamine (Transderm Scp®): patch for motion sickness. Rx.

Use: Treatment and prevention of motion sickness.

Side Effects: The most frequent adverse reaction was dryness of the mouth. This occurred in about two thirds of patients on drug. A less frequent adverse drug reaction was drowsiness, which occurred in less than one sixth of patients on drug. Transient impairment of eye accommodation, including blurred vision and dilation of the pupils, was also observed.

Precautions: Scopolamine should be used with caution in patients with pyloric obstruction or urinary bladder neck obstruction. Urine retention could occur in the later. Caution should be exercised when administering any antiemetic or antimuscarinic drug to patients suspected of having intestinal obstruction. Transderm Scop should be used with caution in the elderly or in individuals with impaired liver or kidney functions because of the increased likelihood of CNS effects. Caution should be exercised in patients with a history of seizures or psychosis because scopolamine can potentially aggravate both disorders.

Administration: One patch applied to the skin behind the ear every 3 days.

Terbinafine (Lamisil® Cream): topical antifungal cream for skin.

Advantages: Quick response and shorter duration of treatment than other topical antifungals.

Disadvantages: Not well-known, expensive.

Use: Suspected fungal infections such as athlete's foot, jock itch, and ringworm.

Side Effects: Generally limited to hypersensitivity reactions.

Precautions: Hypersensitivity to Terbinifine. Do not use for more than 2 weeks. For external use only. Do not use near eyes or for vaginal infections.

Administration: Apply twice a day for maximum of 10 days. Do not use occlusive dressings.

Tincture of benzoin liquid or swabsticks: astringent, makes skin sticky.

Use: Makes skin sticky for better adhesion of tape, steri-strips, and bioclusive dressings. Good for wet environment. Also will dry and harden blistered areas, but produces marked discomfort when applied.

Side Effects: Local skin irritation if allergy or sensitivity.

Precautions: Stings when allowed into or near open wounds. Be careful and warn your patient.

Application: Apply to area a few minutes before applying adhesive. Let dry.

Addendum for Advanced Practitioners and Bibliography

The notes that follow are intended to provide additional information for advanced practitioners, as well as basic level providers interested in the science behind the subject. The literature of wilderness medicine is spotty at best. What we know about altitude illness, for example, is provided by well-designed basic research and clinical trials. By contrast, there is little if any literature formulating and validating evacuation rules for head injuries. This bibliography offers a selection of articles that the authors believe will support or otherwise illuminate issues surrounding the information included in this text. The references either represent current knowledge or offer tangential evidence for medical practice in the remote context of wilderness or rescue medicine. These latter come from hospital and EMS-based studies. We have included some sources that do not support our opinions. This is a work in progress.

CHAPTER 3: THE PATIENT ASSESSMENT SYSTEM

Knowing that we lack the more sophisticated tools found in traditional clinical settings, it is tempting to find alternative techniques to supplement physical assessments to improve the precision in making an earlier diagnosis. These include variations on how to measure vital signs. Gauging a person's volume status following fluid loses by measuring capillary refill time and postural (orthostatic) changes in pulse rate and blood pressure are two such examples. There are problems with accuracy and usefulness of both of these, due in part to the techniques* used for measuring each. Knowing what pathophysiological condition is being sought is equally important. Is it a problem of volume loss from the intravascular space, dehydration, or both? Even when capillary refill is assessed under relatively controlled conditions, it is far from useful for assessing mild to moderate losses from the intravascular space. Posturals do not fare much better. In fact, they are only good predictors of volume loss if the pulse increases by more than 30 beats/minute, or if severe dizziness occurs making the determination of vital signs essentially impossible. Even a rapid pulse rate when lying supine is apparently not helpful. By the time posturals are useful, it should already be clear that the person is sick. Big net issues like mechanism of injury, vital sign trends, and evacuation challenges are more important and useful criteria.

*Determine the pulse and blood pressure after lying supine for at least 2 minutes. Then repeat them after the person has been standing for 1 minute. Sitting for vital signs between lying and standing compromises the accuracy of the measurements.

McGee S, et al. Is this patient hypovolemic? JAMA 1999;281:1022-1029.

Schringer DL, Baraff L. Capillary refill - Is it a useful predictor of hypovolemic states? Ann Emerg Med 1991;20:601-605.

CHAPTER 4: THE CIRCULATORY SYSTEM

Many people are taught about eight or more forms of shock. All of these are just different names or a combination of volume, vascular, and cardiogenic shock. *Distributive shock* is another way of saying vascular shock. Pericardial tamponade and a large pulmonary thrombembolus are examples of *obstructive shock*, where there is blockage of flow, which, in essence, is a manifestation of volume shock. *Anaphylactic shock* is vascular shock, sometimes with profound volume loss from third-spacing. Depending on the stage, *septic shock* can be a combination of all three.

CHAPTER 5: THE RESPIRATORY SYSTEM

It is common for beginners to focus on respiratory rate while advanced practitioners depend on a stethoscope when doing a respiratory assessment. Both have value, but either can lead to a false sense of security or undue alarm. Sometimes the most important and valuable assessment occurs when you observe patients from 2 meters away. How do they look; is there effort with breathing and if so, when? The person with a fever or who has been exerting himself will breathe quickly without undue effort. A patient who is fatigued and ready to go into arrest will often have a low to normal respiratory rate that is ineffective.

When using a stethoscope, it is valuable to have a system for evaluation. In a way, "I hear junky breath sounds" is descriptive but does not take full advantage of a stethoscope's utility as a diagnostic tool. Try to focus on what you hear and when. Divide adventitial sounds into crackles and wheezes and sub-divide crackles into fine and coarse. Then describe what you hear and when, either on inhalation or exhalation, and note if they clear on coughing or continued breathing. For example, fluid in the alveoli is usually accompanied by fine crackles on inhalation; when the fluid gets into the airways, coarse crackles are noted. A totally clear inspiratory phase eliminates the possibility of pulmonary edema or significant fluid in alveoli. Although the sounds are not diagnostic in themselves, they can be helpful when used in the context of the history and other findings.

Forgacs P. The functional basis of pulmonary sounds. Chest 1978;73:399-405.

Pasterkamp H, et al. Respiratory sounds – Advances beyond the sethoscope. Amer J Resp Crit Care Med 1997;156:974-987.

R.A.L.E. Repository. (www.rale.ca.

CHAPTER 6: THE CENTRAL NERVOUS SYSTEM

We have chosen to use AVPU rather than the ubiquitous Glasgow Coma Scale (GCS). It is interesting to see how the GCS has evolved. Initially, it was designed as a "clinical scale . . . for assessing the depth and duration of impaired consciousness and coma" using verbal and motor ability with eye opening. It has evolved to a supposed objective score used by EMS and hospitals for everything from triage to outcome to decision rules for assessing head injuries. In the original article, the researchers published graphs that represented changes in the three parameters over time rather than an aggregate number or score.

Today we assign a single number or score. There are problems with the GCS when it is applied in the field. It is not easy to remember unless one uses it regularly. To be useful, the patient must be able to hear or know the language of the rescuer.

Questions about it being a reliable and accurate tool have been raised in the literature. As a practical matter, the GCS has no value in making difficult assessments about whether or not to evacuate a person with a TBI. At the high end (15) the GCS has limited discriminatory value. The low end is 3, so even a block of wood is not zero. A person with a GCS of 15 could have a terrible headache, persistent vomiting, and/or irritability. And less than 15 should always be grounds for concern (e.g., only opens eyes on command or confused or does not obey commands but localizes pain). In the current spate of decision rules/instruments, a GCS of 15 on presentation or within 2 hours of the initial assessment, is one of the important criteria for deciding not to do a CT scan of the brain.

Glasgow Coma Scale

Gill MR, et al. Interrater reliability of Glasgow Coma Scale in the Emergency Department. Ann Emerg Med 2004;43:215.

Judd JE, et al. Interrater reliability of criteria used in assessing blunt heady injury patients for intracranial injuries. Acad Emerg Med 2003;10:830.

Teasdale G, Jennett B. Assessment of coma and impaired consciousness: A practical scale. Lancet 1974 July 13;2(7872):81-84.

Wiese MF. British hospitals and different versions of the Glasgow coma scale: Telephone survey. Br Med J 2003;327(7418):782–783.

Post Concussive State

Cantu RC, et al. Overview of concussion consensus statements since 2000. Neurosurgical Focus 2006:21(4):E3 (http://www.aans.org/education/journal/neurosurgical/Oct06/21-4-3-1067.pdf)

Harmon KG. Assessment and management of concussion in sports. Amer Fam Phy 1999;60;887-894 (http://www.aafp.org/afp/990901ap/887.html).

Lovell MR, et al. Recovery from mild concussion in high school athletes. J Neurosurg 2003;98;296.

Head Injury Evaluations: When Should We Worry?

Haydel MJ. Clinical decision instruments for CT scanning in minor head injury (Editorial). JAMA 2005;294:1151-1153.

Mower WR, et al. Developing a decision instrument to guide computed tomographic imaging of blunt head injury patients. J Trauma 2005;59:954-950.

Stiell IG, et al. Comparison of the Canadian CT head rule and the New Orleans criteria in patients with minor head trauma. JAMA 2005;294:1511-1518.

CHAPTER 7: SPINE INJURY

Below the surface of apparent agreement brews a stew of unproven science resulting in substantive differences of opinion. Despite the near-universal application of spine stabilization in trauma, there is no convincing literature to document its utility.

Burton JH, et al. A statewide, prehospital emergency medical service selective patient spine immobilization protocol. Journal of Trauma 2006;51:161-167.

Chan, D, et al. The effect of spinal immobilization on healthy volunteers. Emerg Med Svcs 1994;23:48-51.

Domeier RM, et al. Prospective performance assessment of an out-of-hospital protocol for selective spine immobilization using clinical spine clearance criteria. Annals of Emergency Medicine 2005;46:123-131.

Hauswald M, et al. Out-of-hospital spinal immobilization: Its effect on neurologic injury. Acad Emerg Med 1998;5:214-219.

Hoffman JR, et al. Validity of a set of clinical criteria to rule out injury to the cervical spine in patients with blunt trauma. N Engl J Med 2000;343:94-99.

National Association of Emergency Medical Physicians (NAEMSP) Rural Affairs Committee. Clinical Guidelines for delayed/prolonged transport - spine injury. Prehosp Disaster Med 1993;8:174-178.

Orledge JD, Pepe PE. Out-of-hospital spinal immobilization: Is it really necessary (Commentaries). Acad Emerg Med 1998;5:203-204.

Stiell IG, et al. The Canadian C-spine rule versus the NEXUS low-risk criteria in patients with trauma. N Eng J Med 2003;349:2510-2518.

CHAPTER 8: BASIC AND ADVANCED LIFE SUPPORT

Are clot enhancers worthwhile? This seems to be a hot topic because of the hype in the lay press and advertising around their use in combat. To date, the medical literature has not helped to answer the question about their utility because there are only animal studies of questionable clinical relevance and reviews of field practitioner experience. The 2 most highly touted are zeolite containing (QuikClot®) and those made from chitosan (HemCon® and CitoFlex®). The early generation of zeolite was easily blown around by rotor wash and there was concern about heat production. A reformulated version supposedly produces less heat and has been made into a bead impregnated sponge. Interestingly, chitosan did just the opposite, going from a bandage form to a new granular form. Both do enhance clotting to some degree. Field military experience seems to favor the chitosan but that is based on opinion from field experience and not on hard science. One must always ask, even if it works in the field to stop bleeding, does it make a difference in morbidity and mortality? Are there any complications? The jury is still out.

For now, even in the most dire of circumstances, visualizing a wound and then applying pressure directly on the bleeding site will work in the vast majority of injuries in the civilian world. Combat situations may require tourniquets, and yes, maybe even clot enhancers, especially when a field medic must confront multiple casualties and/or multiple seriously bleeding wounds while also contending with hostile fire.

Ahuja N, et al. Testing of modified zeolite hemostatic dressing in a large animal model of lethal groin injury. Journal of Trauma 2006;61: 1312-1320.

Alanzei K, et al. Survival rates for adult trauma patients who require cardiopulmonary resuscitation. Can J Emerg Med 2004;6:263-265.

Cone DC, et al. "The safety of a field termination-of-resuscitation protocol." Prehosp Emerg Care 2005;9:276-281.

Hazinski MF, et al. Major changes in the 2005 AHA Guidelines for CPR ands ECC. Circulation 2005;112:IV-206-211.

National Association of Emergency Medical Physicians (NAEMSP) Rural Affairs Committee. Clinical Guidelines for delayed/prolonged transport - cardiorespiratory arrest. Prehosp Disaster Med 1991;6:335-340.

Pickens JJ, et al. Trauma Patients Receiving CPR: Predictors of Survival. J Trauma 2005;58:951-958.

Stiell IG, et al. Advanced cardiac life support in out-of-hospital arrest. N Engl J Med 2004;351:647-656.

Wedmore I, et al. A Special Report on the Chitosan-based Hemostatic Dressing: Experience in Current Combat Operations.

The entire 2005 AHA/ILCOR document is available online at:
(http://circ.ahajournals.org/content/vol112/22_suppl/).

CHAPTER 9: ALLERGY AND ANAPHYLAXIS

Is it safe for basic providers to administer epinephrine for the treatment of anaphylaxis? The simple answer is yes. In some of the reports purporting to document serious reactions, the epinephrine was administered intravenously. In others, the possibility of an alternative cause was not excluded. We know, for example, that chemicals released during anaphylaxis can cause myocardial dysfunction including dysrhythmia and ischemia. Hypoxia can occur as a result of respiratory involvement. The risks of anaphylaxis make the concerns about the relative contraindications moot in all but a few patients.

Administering epinephrine to any person taking a beta-blocker, including topicals for glaucoma, is a legitimate concern. The unopposed alpha stimulation can lead to worsening bronchospasm and increased coronary artery constriction. These medications can also blunt the normal response to an allergic reaction. If there is concern, the recommendation is to give half the usual dose of epinephrine along with full doses of all of the other drugs.

To our knowledge, no one has demonstrated that any antihistamine is superior to diphenhydramine as an adjunct in the treatment of anaphylaxis. The addition of an H-2 blocker (e.g., famotidine) may be helpful for a particularly bad episode.

AAAI Board of Directors. The use of epinephrine in the treatment of anaphylaxis (Position Statement). J Allergy Clin Immunol 1994;94:666-668.

Davis JE. Allergies and anaphylaxis: Analyzing the spectrum of clinical manifestations. Emerg Med Practice 2005;7:1-24.

Cone DC. Subcutaneous epinephrine for out-of-hospital treatment of anaphylaxis (Position Paper). Prehosp Emerg Care 2002;6:67-68.

Korenblat P, et al. A retrospective study of epinephrine administration for anaphylaxis: How many doses are needed? Allergy Asthma Proc 1999;20:383-386.

Liberman P, et al (eds). The diagnosis and management of anaphylaxis: An updated practice parameter. J Allergy Clin Immunol 2005;115(3, Supplement 2):S465-528. [Note this is a remarkably comprehensive review that can be viewed in its entirety at www.jcaai.org/PP/anaph_toc.asp.]

McLean-Tooke APC, et al. Adrenaline in the treatment of anaphylaxis: What is the evidence. Br Med J 2003;327:1332-1335.

Mrvos R, et al. Accidental injection of epinephrine from an autoinjector: Invasive treatment not always required. S Med J 2002;95:318-320.

Reisman RE. Natural history of insect sting allergy: Relationship of severity of symptoms of initial sting anaphylaxis to resting reactions. J Allergy Clin Immunol 1992;90:335-339.

Sicherer SF, et al. Quandaries in prescribing an emergency action plan and self-injectable epinephrine for first-aid management of anaphylaxis in the community. J Allergy Clin Immunol 2005 ;115:575-583

Toogood JH. Risk of anaphylaxis in patients receiving beta-blocker drugs. J Allergy Clin Immunol 1988;81:1-5.

CHAPTER 10: ASTHMA

Asthma has become a relatively commonly recognized preexisting medical problem in participants in wilderness-based programs. Although inhaled -agonist have revolutionized the treatment of acute exacerbations, treatment with an MDI may be ineffective when a patient is severely short of breath or has an abnormal mental state due to the hypoxia of respiratory failure. Epinephrine, once our only available acute treatment, offers a reasonably safe choice in a remote setting until ALS arrives or transport can be accomplished.

Barnes PJ, Adcock IM. How do steroids work in asthma? Ann Intern Med 2003;139:359-70.

Cydulka R, et al. The use of epinephrine in the treatment of older asthmatic patients. Ann Emerg Med 1988;17:322-326.

Linbeck GH, et al. Out-of-hospital provider use of epinephrine for allergic reactions: Pilot program. Acad Emerg Med 1995;2:592-596.

Rea TD, et al. Epinephrine use by emergency medical technicians for presumed anaphylaxis. Prehosp Emerg Care 2004;8:405-410.

Roberts JR. Epinephrine for the treatment of asthma. Emerg Med News 2005; April: 39-42.

CHAPTER 12: GENERAL PRINCIPLES OF TRAUMA

Initial ALS field treatment for volume shock has traditionally focused on the use of isotonic crystalloids for volume replacement to maintain normal blood pressure. Over the last decade, we have learned how dangerous this approach can be. Large amounts of fluids without cells, protein, or coagulation factors can lead to reduced oxygen carrying capacity of blood and ultimately to coagulopathy and accelerated bleeding. The evolving alternative approach is to administer fluids judiciously. Called permissive hypotension, fluids are administered in volumes sufficient to maintain adequate perfusion. The military monitors radial pulses and uses their presence as a sign of adequate perfusion. This approach, along with monitoring for changes in mental status, would seem to be even more important for evacuations from remote settings.

A corollary to this approach is to substitute hypertonic saline for isotonic crystalloids, taking advantage of a higher effective volume expansion while administering a smaller actual volume. Hypertonic saline continues to be looked at as a substitute. It has yet to find a home. With smaller volumes, it could find a place in the management of ongoing bleeding when transport times will be prolonged.

Bickell WH, et al. Immediate versus delayed fluid resuscitation for hypotensive patients with penetrating torso injuries. N Eng J Med 1994;331:1105-1109.

Gentilello LM, Pierson DJ. Update in nonpulmonary critical care - trauma critical care. Amer J Respir Crit Care Med 2001;163:604-607.

Holcomb JB, et al. Manual vital signs reliably predict need for life-saving interventions in trauma patients. J Trauma 2005;59:821-829.

Revell M, et al. Endpoint for fluid resuscitation of hemorrhagic shock. J Trauma 2002;54:S63-S67.

Sever MS, et al. Management of crush-related injuries after disasters. N Eng J Med 2006;354:1052-1063.

Shafi S, et al. Is hypothermia simply a marker of shock and injury severity or an independent risk factor for mortality in trauma patients? Analysis of a large national trauma registry. J Trauma 2005;59:1081-1085.

Tisherman SA. Regardless of origin, uncontrolled hemorrhage is uncontrolled hemorrhage. Crit Care Med 2000;28:893-895.

CHAPTER 13: MUSCULOSKELETAL INJURY

There is a consensus that some form of pelvic binding is an important and relatively safe way to package a suspected pelvic fracture patient for transport. Traction splints are another issue. Although we argue that their utility is questionable and that they are risky to use on long-term transports, we have included references that argue both sides of the issue.

Pelvic Fractures

Bottlang M, et al. Emergent management of pelvic ring fractures by circumferential compression. J of Bone & Joint Surg 2002;84-A:2, 43-47.

Demetriades D, et al. Pelvic fractures: Epidemiology and predictors of associated abdominal injuries and outcomes. J Am Coll of Surgeons 2002;195:1, 1-9.

Gonzalez P, et al. The utility of clinical examination in screening for pelvic fractures in blunt trauma. J Am Coll of Surgeons 2002;194:2, 121-125.

Ramzy AI, et al. The pelvic sheet wrap. JEMS 2003;5;68-78.

Simpson T, et al. Stabilization of pelvic ring disruptions with a circumferential sheet. J Trauma 2002;52:1, 158-161.

Traction Splints

Abarbanell NR. Prehospital mid thigh trauma and traction splint use: Recommendations for treatment protocols. Am J Emerg Med 2001;19:137-140.

Bledsoe B. Traction splint, An EMS relic? JEMS 2004;29:64-69.

Brown LH, Criss FA. Traction splints in EMS: Don't jump the gun. JEMS 2004;29:69-70.

Kirkup J. Fracture care of friend and foe during WW I. ANZ J Surg 2003;73:453-459.

Mihalko WM, et al. Transient peroneal nerve palsies from injuries placed in traction splints. Am J Emerg Med 1999;17:160-162.

Watson AD, Kelikian AS. Thomas splint, calcaneus fracture, and compartment syndrome of the foot: A case report. J Trauma 1998;44:205-208.

Wood SP, et al: Femur fracture immobilization with traction splints in multisystem trauma patients. Prehosp Emerg Care 2003;7:241-243.

CHAPTER 14: JOINT DISLOCATIONS

Classically, we have been taught that injuries requiring shoulder stabilization should include a sling and swath. This conventional wisdom has been challenged with regard to the post reduction management of an anterior glenohumeral (shoulder) dislocation. Increasingly, the literature suggests that the arm should be splinted so that the shoulder is externally rotated with the forearm pointing out from the body at more than 90°. Why is this? When a shoulder dislocates, the supporting structures of the joint itself – the labrum and the joint capsule –are damaged. Internal rotation exaggerates that disruption. Several studies have shown that external rotation better aligns the structures. In at least one small clinical study, fewer recurrent dislocations occurred when this principle was applied. Hold your arm in full internal rotation and at 90° to your body and you can feel a difference in the tension on the joint.

A major problem with this approach is compliance. It is not simple to walk around with one's arm pointing out from one's body, especially in the backcountry. A compromise would be to get rid of the swathe and keep the forearm angled away from the body by using some padding. You can learn how to make a fancy version of the splint at: www.ori.org.au/bonejoint/shoulder/ssfd/splint.mov

Doyle WL, Ragar T. Use of scapular manipulation method to reduce an anterior shoulder dislocation in the supine position. Ann Emerg Med 1996;27:92-94.

Funkl. How to immobilize after shoulder dislocation? Emergency Medicine Journal 2005 (best evidence topic reports);22:814-815.

Murrell GA. For debate: Treatment of shoulder dislocation: is a sling appropriate? Medical Journal of Australia 2003; 179:370-371.

National Association of Emergency Medical Physicians (NAEMSP) Rural Affairs Committee. Clinical Guidelines for delayed/prolonged transport - dislocations. Prehosp Disaster Med 1993;8:77-80.

Shourkry K, Riou B. Anterior dislocation of shoulder: Reduction in the emergency department without analgesia by scapular rotation and humeral rotation. Ann Int Med 2004;44 (supplement):S128.

CHAPTER 15: WOUNDS AND BURNS

Emergency departments are noting that methicillin resistant *Staphylococcus aureus* (MRSA) is becoming a more frequently identified causative agent for skin infections. Once the scourge of ICUs, chronically ill patients, and persons in jail, MRSA has found its way into healthy patient populations. A unique community-acquired form of MRSA (CA-MRSA) is a major concern because now commonly occurring skin infections are increasingly becoming resistant to previously effective antibiotics. Although we are not aware of any outbreaks in camps or on wilderness trips, it is only a matter of time before they will.

CA-MRSA infections differ from their hospital-based cousins in two important ways. First, they respond to antibiotics other than the expensive choices used in hospitals like vancomycin, linezolid, and daptomycin. Trimethaprim/sulfamethoxazole (TMP/SMX), doxycycline, and clindamycin are three good examples of currently effective alternatives. Depending on the community, some extended coverage flouroquinolones (e.g., leveofloxacin) are effective as well. But like MRSA, none of the usual ß-lactamase antibiotics work and even the ever-popular third generation cephalosporin, ceftriaxone, is ineffective.   Secondly, CA-MRSA infections are currently less likely to represent life-threatening conditions.

The close quarters, mixed populations, wide-ranging travel, and recurrent skin injuries with open sores so common on remote wilderness trips would seem to hold some risk for CA-MRSA. As is always true, effective personal hygiene, good wound care, and completing doses of antibiotics help to decrease the risk for any closed group.

CA-MRSA should be considered the causative agent of a skin infection when there has been a problem with recurrent skin infections, repeated antibiotic use, spread of skin infections within a group, or an invasive case of cellulitis. Also be wary of an alleged brown recluse spider bite when the spider has not been seen and you are not in a known *reclusa* habitat. If you do suspect a CA-MRSA infection, incise and drain any abscesses appropriately, keep open wounds clean and covered, properly dispose of contaminated materials, and choose an effective antibiotic if indicated. Some people have advocated using nasal mupirocin to help control spread by eliminating CA-MRSA carriage until the infections are clear.

Bansal BC, et al. Tap water for irrigation of lacerations. Am J Emerg Med 2002;20:469-472.

Community-associated MRSA information for the public. From The Centers for Disease Control and Prevention 2005. (http://www.cdc.gov/ncidod/dhqp/ar_mrsa_ca_public.html).

Dire DJ, et al. A comparison of wound irrigation solutions used in the emergency department. Ann Emerg Med 1990;19:704-708.

Gravett A, et al. A trial of povidone-iodine in the prevention of infection in sutured lacerations.   Ann Emerg Med 1987;16:167-171.

Moran GJ, Talan DA. Community-acquired methicillin-resistant *Staphylococcus aureus*: Is it in your community and should it change your practice? Ann Emerg Med 2005;45:321-322.

National Association of Emergency Medical Physicians (NAEMSP) Rural Affairs Committee. Clinical Guidelines for delayed/prolonged transport - wounds. Prehosp Disaster Med 1993;8:253-255.

Palacecino E.   Community-acquired methicillin-resistant *Staphylococcus aureus* infections.   Clin Lab Med 2004;24:403-418.

Singer AJ, et al. Pressure Dynamics of Various Irrigation Techniques Commonly Used in the Emergency Department. Ann Emerg Med 1994;24:36-40.

Valente JH, et al. Wound irrigation in children: Saline solution or tap water? Ann Emerg Med 2003;41(5):609-616.

Vonhof J. Fixing your feet. Footwork Publishing, 2000.

CHAPTER 16: THERMOREGULATION

Not everyone agrees on the definition of the different levels of hypothermia. Mild hypothermia is a depressed body temperature with shivering and an impaired mental state confirmed by a core temperature between 35 to 32°C. Moderate/severe is below that temperature, characterized by no shivering and/or loss of consciousness. People at this level are at increased risk for a lethal cardiac dysrhythmia. Some experts further subdivide these levels, noting that shivering stops between 32 to 28°C, loss of conscious occurs at 28 to 24°C, and breathing ceases below 24°C. For field treatment, the clinical transition from when shivering stops or loss of consciousness occurs is what matters for treatment.

Treatment with many medications can make a person more susceptible to environmental stressors by impairing the body's normal thermoregulatory response to either a cold or heat challenge. These effects can be central, peripheral, or a combination of the two. Sometimes the mechanism is unclear. Medication use should be a prescreening as well as an in-field treatment consideration.

There are several mechanisms to consider in cold environments. Vascular dilation with concomitant increased heat loss can be caused by antihypertensives (e.g., clonidie) and narcotic pain medications (e.g., morphine, meperidine). Heat production is decreased when shivering is depressed by narcotic pain medication, paralytics (e.g., succinylcholine and vecuronium), sedatives in the benzodiazepine family (e.g., lorazepam), and -blockers (e.g., propranolol, metropolol). Lithium suppresses thyroid function and diuretics deplete fluid volume. Antipsychotic medications like risperidone and olanzapine have reportedly been associated with hypothermia. Because of their complex pharmacology, any of several mechanisms could be responsible. It would not be surprising if these medications also made their users more susceptible to heat related conditions.

Heat susceptibility can be caused by anticholinergic effects, increased adrenergic stimulation, and volume depletion. Many medications have anticholinergic effects, including antipsychotics, some antidepressants, and over-the-counter antihistamines. Anticholinergic effects include decreased sweating, diminished gastrointestinal absorption, dehydration, impaired central thermoregulation, and motor restlessness. Adrenergic stimulation can be caused by direct stimulation and direct or indirect increase in norepinephrine. Over-the-counter decongestants, stimulants used for ADHD (e.g., methylphenidate), methamphetamines and cocaine, and antidepressants, including tricyclics and MAO inhibitors, can be included here. People on these medications are at an even higher risk of heat related problems when they are unacclimatized and working in a hot environment. This is particularly worrisome because many of these drugs are so commonly used. Malignant hyperthermia is a separate entity.

Cold
Gentilello LM, et al. Continuous arteriovenous rewarming: Rapid reversal of hypothermia in critically ill patients. J Trauma 1992;32:316-327.

Giesbrecht GG. Cold stress, near drowning and accidental hypothermia: A review. Aviat Space Environ Med 2000;71:733-752.

Giesbrecht GG. Prehospital treatment of hypothermia. Wilderness Environ Med 2001;12(1):24-31.

Gilbert M, et al. Resuscitation from accidental hypothermia of 13.7°C with circulatory arrest. Lancet 2000;355:375–376.

Kornberger E, et al. Forced air surface rewarming in patients with severe accidental hypothermia. Resuscitation 1999;41:105–111.

Robinaon J, et al. Oesophageal, rectal, axillary, tympanic and pulmonary artery temperatures during cardiac surgery. Can J Anaesth 1998;45:317-323.

Silfvast T, Pettila V. Outcome from severe accidental hypothermia in Southern Finland—a 10-year review. Resuscitation 2003;59:285–290.

State of Alaska Cold Injuries Guidelines. (www.chems.alaska.gov/EMS/documents/AKColdInj2005.pdf).

Hot
Almond CSD, et al. Hyponatremia among runners in the Boston Marathon. N Engl J Med 2005;352:1550.

Bouchama A, Knochel JP. Heat stroke. N Engl J Med 2002;346:1978-1988.

Cheung SS, et al. The thermophysiology of uncompensable heat stress. Sports Med 2000;29:329-359.

Collins S, Reynolds B. The other heat-related emergency. JEMS 2004; 29:75-88.

Dematte JE, et al. Near-fatal heat stroke during the 1995 heat wave in Chicago. Ann Int Med 1998;129:173-181.

Martinez M. Drug-associated heat stroke. S Med J 2002;95:799-802.

Noakes TD. International Marathon Medical Directors Association Advisory Statement on Guidelines for Fluid Replacement During Marathon Running. November 2001.

Valtin H."Drink at least eight glasses of water a day." Really? Is there scientific evidence for "8 × 8"? Am J Physiol Regulation Integrative Comparative Physiology 2002;993-1004.

Various authors. Features and outcomes of classic heat stroke. Ann Int Med 1999;130:613-615 (letters to ed).

Yeo TP. Heat stroke: A comprehensive review. AACN Clinical Issues 2004;15:280-293.

CHAPTER 17: COLD INJURIES

Despite the occasional article to the contrary and until substantial proof can be offered, Dr. William Mills' approach is still unchallenged. Based on his experience with hundreds of patients, the emphasis should be focused on good wound care and patience.

Cauchy E, et al. Retrospective study of 70 cases of severe frostbite lesion: A proposed new classification scheme. Wilderness Environ Med 2001;12:248-255.

Harichi I, et al. Frostbite: incidence and predisposing factors in mountaineers. British SportsJournal 2005;39:898-901.

Koljonen V, et al. Frostbite injuries treated in the Helsinki area from 1995-2002. J Trauma 2004;57:1315-1320.

State of Alaska Cold Injuries Guidelines. (www.chems.alaska.gov/EMS/documents/AKColdInj2005.pdf).

CHAPTER 18: ALTITUDE ILLNESS

How does acetazolamide work? As a carbonic anhydrase inhibitor, acetazolimide has two potentially useful effects at altitude. First, it slows the hydration of carbon dioxide which in turn increases the excretion of bicarbonate in the kidneys. This effect begins within 1 hour of ingestion. As a result, the alkalosis caused by hyperventilation is balanced by the creation of a more acidic milieu. The net result is continued ventilatory stimulation that minimizes sleep hypoxia brought on by pH related apnea. Acetazolamide also decreases the production of cerebrospinal fluid. Theoretically, this may help to ameliorate symptoms resulting from brain swelling, particularly in AMS.

That it works to prevent and treat AMS is not in dispute. There is question about its utility once HAPE and HACE are clearly established. The optimal dosage regimen is in question as well. The answer to the former is not so clear to me, but it is probably little if any. Certainly we have other stronger medication for acute deterioration. Although some advocate for a higher dose, 125–250 mg twice/day seems to work best.

Bartsch P, et al. Physiological aspects of high-altitude pulmonary edema. J of Appl Physiol 2005;98:1101-1110.

Basynyat B, Murdoch DR. High altitude illness. Lancet 2003;361:1967-1974.

Dumont L, et al. Efficacy and harm of pharmacological prevention of acute mountain sickness: Quantitative systematic review. B Med J 2000;321:267-272.

Ghofrani HA, et al. Sildenafil increased exercise capacity during hypoxia at low altitudes and at Mount Everest Base Camp. Ann Intern Med 2004;141:169-177.

Hackett PH, Roach RC. High-altitude illness. N Engl J Med 2001;345:107-113.

Hackett PH, et al. High-altitude cerebral edema evaluated with magnetic resonance imaging. JAMA 1998;280:1920-1925.

Maggiorini M, et al. Both tadalafil and dexamethasone may reduce the incidence of high-altitude pulmonary edema: a randomized trial. Annals of InternalMedicine 2006;145:497-506.

Neumann K. Children at high altitude. Wilderness Med Letter 2002;19:1-6.

Niermeyer S. The pregnant altitude visitor. Adv Exp Med Biol 1999;474:65-77.

Sartori C, et al. Salmeterol for the prevention of high-altitude pulmonary edema. N Eng J Med 2002;346:1631-1636.

West JB. The physiologic basis of high-altitude diseases. Ann Int Med 2004;141:789-800.

Chapter 19: Medical Aspects of Avalanche Rescue

Brugger H, Durrer B. On site treatment of avalanche victims. In: Elsensohn F (ed). Consensus Guidelines on Mountain Emergency Medicine and Risk Reduction. ICAR-MEDCOM 2001.

Falk M, et al. Calculation of survival as a function of avalanche burial. Wilderness Environ Med 2001;12:140-141.

Grissom CK, et al. Hypercapnia increases core temperature cooling rate during snow burial. J Appl Physiol 2004;96{1365-1370.

Johnson SM, et al. Avalanche trauma and closed head injury: Adding insult to injury. Wilderness Environ Med 2001;12:244-247.

Radwin MI, et al. Normal oxygenation and ventilation during snow burial by the exclusion of carbon dioxide exclusion. Wilderness Environ Med 2001;12:256-262.

Radwin MI, et al. Technological advances in avalanche survival. Wilderness Environ Med 2002;13:143-152.

State of Alaska Cold Injuries Guidelines. (www.chems.alaska.gov/EMS/documents/AKColdInj2005.pdf).

CHAPTER 20: SUBMERSION INJURY

How long can someone be submersed and still survive? The longest known survivor reported in the literature was a 2½-year-old child believed to have been submersed for 66 minutes in 5°C water. Her rectal temperature on arrival in the hospital was 22.4°C.   The resuscitation included immediate CPR and airway management by an ALS unit in the field and continued ALS support with extracorporeal rewarming by bypass with a membrane oxygenator in the hospital. There have been others more recently, but none so long. Cummings and Quan's report from Kings County, Washington, would seem to suggest that this was an exceptional case. They found that the probability of survival for an under 20-year-old population in water more than 5° C was essentially zero when the patient had been submersed for more than 25 minutes, was in complete arrest at the time of arrival in the emergency department, or CPR continued for more than 25 minutes. In looking at the same population from the mid-1970s to the mid-1990s, they noted no improvement in survivability that could be attributable to advances in medical care.   If we can believe conventional wisdom, adults would fair no better. Perhaps this is why we are not seeing survivors of longer submersion.

Is there any way to predict which submersion patients will develop delayed pulmonary edema? Pathophysiologically, it seems that it is related to brain ischemia and aspiration of water. Therefore, unless the person loses consciousness, this complication is unlikely. Szpilman looked at complications following submersions and developed a classification scheme based on the on-scene evaluations utilizing vital signs and lungs sounds. Essentially, if the person's lung sounds were clear (Grade 1), mortality was zero. Even with localized crackles and a normal blood pressure (Grade 2), the mortality was less than 1%. Interestingly, a normal or near-normal mental state was predictive of a good outcome; the need for positive pressure ventilations was bad.

Bolte RG, et al. The use of extracorporeal rewarming in a child submerged for 66 minutes. JAMA 1988;260:377-379.

Cummings P, Quan L. Trends in unintentional drowning: The role of alcohol and medical care. JAMA 1999;281:2198-2202.

Modell JH, et al. Survival after prolonged submersion in freshwater in Florida. Chest 2004;125:1948-1952.

Quan L, Kinder D. Pediatric submersions: Prehospital predictors of outcome. Pediatrics 1992;90:909-913.

Szpilman D. Near-drowning and drowning classification - a proposal to stratify mortality based on the analysis of 1,831 cases. Chest 1997;112:660-665.

CHAPTER 21: SCUBA DIVING INJURIES

Moon RR, Shefffield PJ. Guidelines for treatment of decompression illness. Aviat Space Environ Med 1997;68:234-242.

CHAPTER 22: LIGHTNING INJURIES

Carte AE, et al. A large group of children struck by lightning. Ann Emerg Med 2002;39:665-70.

Cooper MA. Emergent care of lightning and electrical injuries. Sem in Neuro 1995;15:268-78.

Cooper MA. A fifth mechanism of lightning injury. Acad Emerg Med 2002;9:172-4

Cooper MA. Myths, miracles and mirages. Sem in Neuro 1995;15:358-61.

Zimmerman C, et al. Lightning safety guidelines. Ann Emerg Med 2002;39:660-664 (From the Lightning Safety Group.)

CHAPTER 23: TOXINS

Please note that our efforts to date here are almost exclusively weighted toward problems in the Western Hemisphere and North America, in particular. We are working to change this apparent provincialism by expanding the scope in future editions of this text.

Only honeybees leave their stingers behind, eviscerating and thus killing themselves after only one sting. The conventional wisdom is that if it is stuck in a victim's skin, it should be scraped off rather then pulled out for fear of squeezing the venom sac and therefore more toxin into the sting victim. It turns out that pulling the stinger out with one's fingers has no effect on the reaction and scraping can actually break the stinger off, leaving part of it in the skin. In general, the longer the stinger is left in (up to 8 seconds), the greater the reaction. Remove it any way that you can.

Although relatively infrequent, brown recluse spider bites can cause significant necrotic skin lesions that may ultimately require skin grafting. Lesions attributable to such bites are over diagnosed. In fact, *bites* with subsequent lesions are reported in areas of North American where a brown recluse has never been spotted. As it turns out, their range is concentrated in the south-central part of the United States. Still, there are clinicians who will argue that they have seen brown recluse bites in areas outside the spider's known habitat. Some have attributed the bites to *hitchhikers* that may have come from one area to another by way of car or truck. As our climate warms, the range of insects, spiders and other arthropods is changing. Still, these factors cannot account for the number that occur where they should not.

The main problem of misdiagnosing one of these lesions is that the real diagnosis, such as CA-MRSA (see above under wounds) or cutaneous anthrax, may be overlooked, resulting in the delay of appropriate treatment and the potential spread to other people. Another problem is inappropriate treatment. Although research has failed to convincingly demonstrate that any medications or modalities are effective to treat a brown recluse bite, people are still using some of them. Using a potentially harmful treatment could magnify the harm of not treating the right problem. Particularly in an area not known as a brown recluse habitat, most experts recommend that the alleged offending spider should be positively identified before diagnosing such a bite. Wound cultures are definitely indicated as well.

Except in North America, a compression wrap is the treatment of choice for many snake envenomations. The theory is that the wrap will impede migration of the toxin proximally thus slowing the onset of symptoms until antivenom can be administered. Based on or at least prompted by a 2005 article in the Annals of Emergency Medicine, there seems to be renewed interest in the potential utility of this technique as a field treatment for envenomations from North America's only indigenous elapid, the coral snake or *Micrurus fulvis fulvius*.

The technique involves circumferentially wrapping the envenomated limb with a bandage, starting either at the bite site or at its most distal portion and progressing as far proximally as possible. If the area is covered by a shirt or slacks, the wrap is supposed to be applied over the clothing. The tension should be applied as firmly as an ankle wrap, so that it will be comfortable for several hours. Howarth et al believed that the optimal pressure should be between 40 – 70 mm Hg for the upper and 55 – 70 mm Hg in the lower limb. The limb should then be splinted to restrict movement.

Is this justified? German et al suggest that it works. Norris et al demonstrated that even when prompted by written material detailing how to perform the technique, the wrap was often applied improperly. Howarth et al believe the technique to be ineffective if applied improperly. Further, some believe that Howarth et al's results indicate that improper application (i.e., either too tight or not tight enough) can actually increase venom migration. In general, the literature addressing the utility and efficacy of compression wraps is represented by case studies and small trials using either an animal model or humans injected with a mock venom.

What should we do? Learn and practice the technique if you are going to Australia, Southeast Asia or other places where you will be outdoors and potentially exposed to highly toxic elapids. If you live in the Southeast United States and have not learned the technique yet, forgive yourself. Death from a coral snake envenomation is very rare. In fact, with the possible exception of 2006, there has not been a death from one for about 40 years. By the way, there is no current literature endorsing this technique for pit viper envenomations.

Alberts MB, et al. Suction for venomous snakebite: A study of "mock venom" extraction in a human model. Ann Emerg Med 2004;43:181.

Dart RC, McNally J. Efficacy, safety and use of snake antivenoms in the United States. Ann Emerg Med 2001;37:181-188.

German BT, et al. Pressure-immobilization bandages delay toxicity in a porcine model of Eastern coral snake (*Micrurus fulvis fulvius*) envenomation. Ann Emerg Med 2005;45:603-608.

Gold BS, et al. Bites of venomous snakes. N Eng J Med 2002;347:347-356.

Howarth DM, et al. Lymphatic flow rates and first aid in simulated peripheral snake or spider envenomation. Med J Aust 1994;161:695-700.

Norris RL, et al. Physicians and lay people are unable to apply pressure immobilization properly in a simulated snakebite scenario. Wilderness Environ Med 2005;16:16-21.

Isbister GK, Kiernan MC. Neurotoxic marine poisoning. Lancet Neurol 2005;4:219-228.

Swanson DL, Vetter R. Bites of brown recluse spiders and suspected necrotic arachnidism. N Eng J Med 2005;352:700-707.

Tokish JT, et al. Crotalid envenomation: the Southern Arizona experience. J of Orthop Trauma 2001;15:5-9.

The University of Melbourne. Pressure-immobilisation first aid for venomous bites and stings Available at: http:// www.avru.unimelb.edu.au/avruweb/pi.htm.

Various authors. Bites of venomous snakes. N Eng J Med 2002;347:1804-1805.

Warrell DA. Treatment of bites by adders and exotic venomous snakes. BMJ 2005;331:1244-1247.

CHAPTER 24: ARTHROPOD DISEASE VECTORS

Insect repellents containing DEET continue to be the gold standard against which others are measured. DEET is remarkably safe and effective when used in concentrations to the low 30% range. Some of the newer formulations use vehicles that make them more resilient to the environment. The result is that they are less likely to be absorbed and require fewer applications. Picardin is a newer ingredient that has been available around the world for several years and in the United States since 1995. Besides being odorless and plastic friendly, it is an attractive alternative because it is as effective as DEET at comparable concentrations. For now, however, it is only available in the United States in concentrations less than 20%. Both ingredients are effective against ticks and mosquitoes. Really effective tick protection, however, requires supplemental measures and surveillance. The CDC also recognizes lemon/eucalyptus-based repellents as an alternative. This type is much less effective against mosquitoes, not proven against malaria, and not effective against ticks.

Centers for Disease Control. West Nile Virus Home (http://www.cdc.gov/ncidod/dvbid/westnile/index.htm).

Edlow JA. Lyme disease and related tick-borne illnesses. Ann Emerg Med 1999;33:680-693.

Felz MW, et al. A six-year-old girl with tick paralysis. N Eng J Med 2000;342:90-94.

Fradin MS. Mosquitoes and mosquito repellents: A clinicians' guide. Ann Inten Med 1998;128:931.

Fradin MS, Day JF. Comparative Efficacy of Insect Repellents against Mosquito Bites. N Eng J Med 2002;347:13.

McQuiston, JH, et al. The human ehrlichioses in the United States (Synopses). Emerg Infect Dis 1999;5:635-642.

Nadelman RB, Nowakowski J, Fish D, et al. Prophylaxis with single-dose doxycycline for the prevention of lyme disease after an ixodes scapularis tick bite. N Eng J Med 2001;345:79-84.

Picardin. A new insect repellent. Medical Letter 6 June 2005;47(1210):46.

Shapiro ED. Doxycycline for tick bites—not for everyone (editorial). N Engl J Med. 2001;345:133-134.

Steere AC. Lyme Disease. N Eng J Med 2001;345:115-125.

Visscher PK, et al. Removing bee stings. Lancet 1996;348:301-302.

CHAPTER 25: AN APPROACH TO ILLNESS

Grocott MPW, et al. Resuscitation from hemorrhagic shock using rectally administered fluids in a wilderness environment. Wilderness Environ Med 2005;16:209-211.

Mange K, et al. Language guiding therapy: The case of dehydration versus volume depletion. Ann Int Med 1997;127:848-853.

Sasson M, Shvartzman P. Hypodermolclysis: An alternative infusion technique. Amer Fam Phy 2001;64:1575-1578.

Sudeep G, et al. Hypodermoclysis in the treatment of dehydration (editorial). Am Fam Phys 2001;64:1516.

Thomas EAH, et al. Drugs and the administration in extreme environments. J of Travel Med 2006;13:35-47.

Yasmin K, Zhanel GG. Floroquinolone-associated tendinopathy: A critical review of the literature. Clin Infect Dis 2003;36:1404-1410.

Acknowledgements

We would like to express our sincere appreciation for the efforts of all of the instructors and staff of Wilderness Medical Associates and WMA Canada. Having a stadium-full of experts to consult with is a rare privilege and a considerable benefit, not to mention a challenge. All of you have contributed to the success of the company and the production of this text and its associated materials. In particular, we would like to thank Cheryl Ahern, Mary Beth Brandt, Doug Cameron, Tom Clausing, Anne Dunphy, Robb Evis, Erik Forsythe, Greg Friese, Judi Gauvreau, Emily Hinman, John Jacobs, Fay Johnson, Becka Kangas, Denis Langlois, Ray Martodam, Christin Moser, Mike Motti, Craig Rees, Anne Rugg, Dugg Steary, Cabot Stone, Mike Webster, and Laura Wininger.

We would also like to thank the Medical Library staff at Central Maine Medical Center for its prompt, accurate, and enthusiastic efforts to find and organize medical reference materials. We sincerely appreciate Drs. Peter Hackett, William Mills, Mary Ann Cooper, Gordon Giesbrecht, and Frank Walter sharing their insight and experience. And, as always, we owe a great debt of gratitude to Dr. Peter Goth for having the wisdom to recognize a good idea and the courage to promote it.

Our appreciation is extended to the Crested Butte Professional Ski Patrol, Crested Butte Search and Rescue, the Crested Butte Medical Center, and the Elk Avenue Medical Center for providing a solid base of practical experience and an unparalleled opportunity to consumer-test protocols, equipment, and technique.

We also wish to acknowledge that the only real way to create a useful text is to respond to the people who are using it. We will be most grateful for any comments and critique from our readers, students, and instructors.

With profound gratitude,

Jeffrey E. Isaac, PA-C and David E. Johnson, MD

About the Authors

Jeffrey E. Isaac is a physician assistant with a particular interest in remote and extreme environments. He is a lead instructor and Curriculum Director for Wilderness Medical Associates. His 30 years of experience in emergency medicine includes service as a firefighter, EMT, professional ski patroller, search and rescue team leader, and medical practitioner in hospital emergency departments and ski area clinics.

Jeff is also a licensed captain and an experienced blue water sailor, having logged thousands of miles in the Atlantic and Pacific Oceans, and the Caribbean Sea. His outdoor resume includes 20 years as an instructor and course director with the Hurricane Island Outward Bound School, as well as numerous treks by foot, horse, and canoe throughout North America.

David E. Johnson is an emergency physician and the owner and president of Wilderness Medical Associates. His experience in trans-Atlantic sailing expeditions, numerous land-based expeditions in North and South America, as well as urban emergency medicine has given him a very broad base of extended patient care in difficult and demanding situations.

David is a frequent conference presenter and author, and has taught all levels of EMS and wilderness medicine courses throughout the US and in some of the more far-flung corners of the world. He is known for being firmly committed to the science behind the subject, as well as its practical application at all levels of medical training. For these efforts, David has been recognized by Outward Bound USA with the McGory Award for outstanding contributions to experiential education.

NOTES:

NOTES:

NOTES: